STEVE

L(BE'

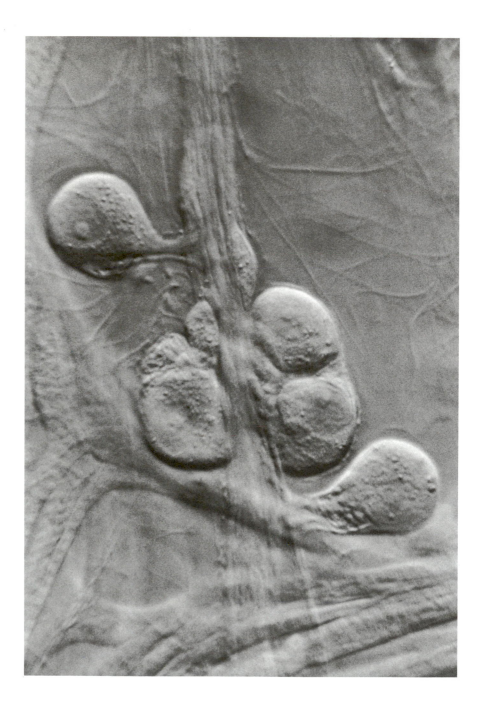

STEVE

Remembrances of Stephen W. Kuffler

Compiled and Introduced

by

U. J. McMahan

Professor and Chairman of Neurobiology
Stanford University School of Medicine

Including a biography by
Sir Bernard Katz

SINAUER ASSOCIATES, INC., PUBLISHERS
Sunderland, Massachusetts

THE COVER

Steve. Photograph by J. Gagliardi.

FRONTISPIECE

Nerve cells and muscle fibers in the isolated septum of the frog's heart photographed by Steve and UJM using Nomarski (DIC) optics (ca. 1968). With this preparation and optics, Steve, along with Mike Dennis and John Harris, mapped for the first time the chemosensitivity of vertebrate nerve cells to neurotransmitter.

The biography by Sir Bernard Katz, which begins on page 108, is reprinted by permission of The Royal Society from *The Biographical Memoirs of Fellows of the Royal Society*, Volume 28, 1982.

STEVE: REMEMBRANCES OF STEPHEN W. KUFFLER
First Printing
Copyright © 1990 by Sinauer Associates Inc.
All rights reserved. For information address
Sinauer Associates, Inc.
Sunderland, Massachusetts 01375, U.S.A.

Library of Congress Cataloging-in-Publication Data

Steve : remembrances of Stephen W. Kuffler / compiled and
    introduced by U. J. McMahan, including a biography by Sir
    Bernard Katz
        p.   cm.
    Includes bibliographical references.
    ISBN 0-87893-516-9 (paper)
    1. Neurophysiology.   2. Kuffler, Stephen W.   I. McMahan,
    U. J.   II. Katz, Bernard, 1911-
    QP355.2.S75   1990
    591.1'88—dc20
    [B]   90-10383
                                                              CIP

Printed in U.S.A.

To Phyllis
and the children:
Suzie, Damien, Genie, and Julian

Contents

PREFACE

Steve Kuffler died ten years ago this month. To scientists who knew him his death has been a deeply felt loss. As a master experimentalist with a broad range of interests in the nervous system he provided crucial leadership for the development of the field of neurobiology, but the lessons he taught by example about how to do research and how to interact with one's students and colleagues transcended specific disciplines, and they are timeless.

I recently interviewed a prospective graduate student for the Neurosciences Ph.D. Program at Stanford. She was doing an undergraduate honors thesis project at another university in the laboratory of a distinguished neurobiologist and had taken an impressive number of neuroscience courses for an undergraduate. She had already interviewed at the Department of Neurobiology at Harvard, and during the course of our conversation, not knowing that I had been in that department and had worked there with Steve, she asked if I had ever heard of Stephen Kuffler. It was a name mentioned often at Harvard, but she hadn't run across it in her studies. She found it hard to believe that all of the stories she had heard about him were true. "Was he really as important as they say?" "Was he really that clever?" "Did all of those famous people work in his department?"

A little later, I visited Ann Stuart, a Harvard colleague of my era, now at the University of North Carolina. I told her the story about the curious undergraduate and we both lamented that less than ten years after his death, the most dominant figure in neuroscience for more than two decades is known only to those who lived through that period. A few days after returning to Stanford I received a letter from Ann asking, since I was close to Steve, whether I would be willing to put together a book portraying his many attributes. At first I completely dismissed the idea because Sir Bernard Katz had already written an excellent biography of Steve for The Royal Society. But as I discussed Ann's suggestion with more and more colleagues, it became evident that few of even Steve's closest friends knew about the biography, and that many of the things that made Steve what he was might be best said in a less formal setting.

This volume is the upshot. I tried to capture Steve in print by presenting a collection of vignettes in the form of letters, each composed by one of his students or colleagues. I am grateful to all those who responded to my request for a letter; in many cases it is clear that writing about Steve was emotionally painful. The letters are unedited. I have merely added material to link and, in some cases, augment them. I am grateful to Sir Bernard Katz and The Royal Society for permitting the inclusion of the biography. Perhaps mistakenly, I did not ask for a letter from Sir Bernard because the biography is an already in-depth exposition. I thank Cecele Thomas for excellent and unfailing assistance in collecting the letters and adapting them for publication. And I am grateful to Andy Sinauer for publishing the book despite the possibility that it may be of narrow appeal. Sinauer Associates published Kuffler and Nicholls' highly successful *From Neuron to Brain* (and the subsequent edition which includes a third author, R. A. Martin). Steve enjoyed his relationship with Andy.

U. J. McMahan
Stanford University
October 1990

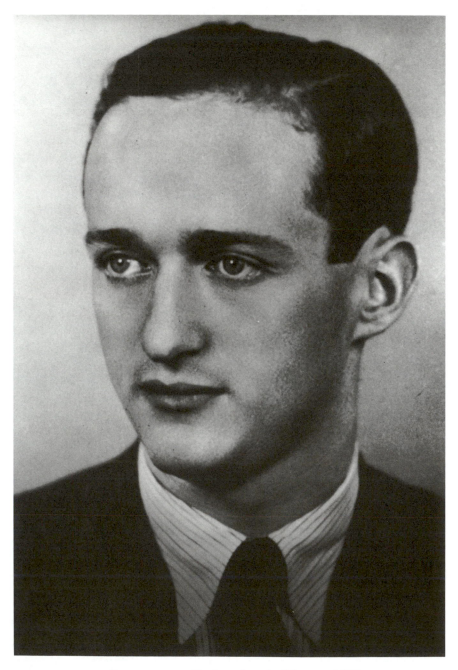

Steve as a medical student in Vienna, 1937.

EARLY DAYS

I began working with Steve in 1967. He was 54 years old. By then he was a full professor at Harvard and, along with David Hubel, Torsten Wiesel, Ed Furshpan, Dave Potter, and Ed Kravitz, he had just formed the Department of Neurobiology. He was chairman, but unlike many of his counterparts then and now he was also an active experimentalist.

Upon my arrival I was already aware of much of his history. It was well known that he did not go to school until the age of 10 or 11, that he trained as a physician in Vienna, that he entered the field of physiology as the result of a chance meeting with John Eccles on a tennis court in Australia in the late 1930s, and that along with Eccles and Bernard Katz, both of whom later became Nobel laureates, he had made important discoveries on the mechanism of neuromuscular transmission. From Australia he had traveled to the University of Chicago to work in the laboratory of Ralph Gerard. Gerard and Gilbert Ling were making the first intracellular microelectrode recordings, a procedure at which Steve became expert. Steve had taken his first independent position in 1947 at the Wilmer Institute, which is associated with Johns Hopkins Medical School, and had moved to Harvard in 1959. His contributions to numerous areas of neuroscience were legendary, and it was apparent to everyone that the top academic positions in the field throughout the world were occupied by his former students.

In 1967 Steve and Phyllis's children were nearing adulthood. Suzie and Damien were away at college (Damien later earned a Ph.D. in Physiology at UCLA and is now a neuroscientist at the Institute of Neurobiology at the University of Puerto Rico). Genie was just leaving to study music in Paris, and Julian was about to graduate from high school. That summer, as in previous ones and ones to come, the family gathered at their huge Victorian house in Newton, a suburb of Boston, to travel to their "real" home at Woods Hole, on Cape Cod, where Steve would do research at the Marine Biological Laboratory (MBL).

The following set of letters provides glimpses of Steve during the early days of his career. Laporte worked with him in Chicago, while Quilliam, Hunt, Eyzaguirre, Trautwein, and Dudel were his first students at the Wilmer.

1

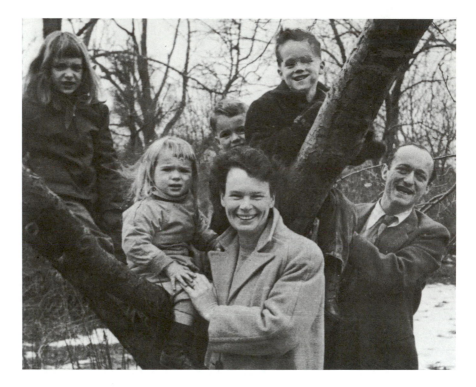

Phyllis and Steve with Suzie, Genie, Julian, and Damien in Baltimore, 1951.

Peter Quilliam

The Chairman (immediate past) of Convocation
Professor Emeritus in Pharmacology
St. Bartholomew's Hospital Medical College
London, United Kingdom

I am delighted to contribute to the volume marking the tenth anniversary of Steve's death. During my 17 years as Chairman of Convocation, I derived the greatest satisfaction when the Honorary Degrees Committee of the Senate recommended to Senate that a Doctorate of Science *Honoris Causa* be conferred on Steve for his brilliant research. The Senate so resolved.

The Public Orator was a theologician and turned to me for help with the citation. This citation is enclosed as delivered on Foundation Day 1974 when Steve was presented to our then Chancellor HM Queen Elizabeth, the Queen Mother, who then conferred the Hon. D Sc upon him. As only about six London Hon. Degrees are conferred annually, this was a signal honour. The citation encapsulates my feelings for "my Master" whose influence was seminal to me as I was on the road to getting up a Department of Pharmacology at Barts geared to electropharmacology. Any success which I and my pupils have had (and 26 now hold chairs, two with FRSs) has stemmed largely from his training, example and inspiration.

The enclosed citation shows the breadth and warmth of this remarkable man.

Introduction to the Queen Mother
From Celebration of Foundation Day
Thursday, 28 November 1974
Orations by the Public Orator
The Rev. Canon S. H. Evans, MA

Your Majesty and Chancellor, I present Professor Stephen Kuffler.

We welcome a distinguished visitor from the other side of the Atlantic. Stephen Kuffler is Professor of Neurophysiology and Neuropharmacology [*sic*] at the Harvard Medical School. Until last year he was head also of the Department of Neurobiology. This means that he's the sort of scientist who specializes in the minute rather than in the massive, and finds electron-microscopes more useful than radio telescopes.

Born in Hungary in 1913 he was educated in Austria at a Jesuit *gymnasium* where he acquired large Latin, less Greek and no Science. Choosing medicine "because of its international character," our Honorary Graduand spent five years in medical school in Vienna at a time of increasing violence and social unrest, specialising in pathology which he regards as the basis of good medicine and earning the money to do so by giving tuition—in Latin and Greek—to high school students whose conjugations were in a state of declension. When Austria was invaded in 1938 Stephen Kuffler made his way to London via Hungary; finding that his medical qualifications were not deemed sufficiently respectable in this country, he bought a ticket for Brisbane but fortuitously left the ship at Sydney. Here his prowess as former junior tennis champion of Austria brought him to the notice of Dr. John Eccles, head of the School of Neurophysiology. With a fine intuition Eccles decided that so apt a tennis player must have the kind of muscular control needed for doing delicate dissections and might even eventually learn some neurophysiology. By the time Bernard Katz from A. V. Hill's Department of Biophysics at University College London arrived to transform a formidable scientific duet into a spectacular trio, Stephen Kuffler had developed his manual skills to an elegance of technique surpassing anything achieved before. Devising his own tools he discovered how to dissect out a single nerve–muscle junction and to make pioneer extracellular recordings from it at an interface between a salt solution and medicinal liquid paraffin. All his subsequent investigations have been characterised by the application of exquisite manual techniques devised to secure results that are surprisingly simplistic.

Practical experience as a consultant neurologist working on nerve injuries suffered by combatants in the war in the Pacific led on to a fellowship in Chicago in 1945–47 and so to what was to become a decade of exceptionally successful scientific co-operation in a small basement laboratory in the Department of Ophthalmology in the Wilmer Institute at Johns Hopkins Medical School, Stephen Kuffler attracted able young men from all over the world. He modestly attributes the productivity of these years to the youthfulness of the group

4

and the benevolent indifference of the authorities. One such young man was a certain Peter Quilliam from our own University.

Our Honorary Graduand, Ma'am, has trained and inspired a whole generation of neurophysiologists and since 1959 there's been almost a shuttle service of able young scientists passing between Sir Bernard Katz at University College and Professor Kuffler at Harvard. For this no less than for his own pioneering we are glad to honour Stephen Kuffler tonight.

His personality has been no less influential than his intellectual distinction in maintaining this high level collaboration. Where Kuffler is, there fun abounds and laughter never flags. An habitual punster, his friends imposed a ban on more than two puns in any one day. But he had other ways of loosening the facial muscles of the overly solemn. The formality of a lecture at an international congress of scientists at Buenos Aires was unstarched when Kuffler received the pendant microphone from the chairman as if he was receiving a medal: in Paris once he pulled out a manuscript and began reading a Spanish translation of a previous lecture: mock consternation: "Oh dear! Wrong country!" A touch of goonery coupled with kindness, the absence of all pretentiousness and the ability to laugh at himself endear him to friends and colleagues alike.

Professor Kuffler, Ma'am, has not been unheard in this country. He gave the Ferrier Lecture to The Royal Society in 1965, the Sherrington Lecture at Liverpool in 1972 and was elected a foreign member of The Royal Society in 1971.

Our Honorary Graduand works at a basic level. He seeks out new approaches to problems and opens up new fields in which others follow up and develop what he has begun. A flair for detecting what's really important is matched by a genius for asking the deceptively simple question that after many hours of patient work yields the answer. Using basically simple preparations Kuffler has discovered mechanisms whereby cells on the retina of the eye receive information; he has elucidated the functions of those mysterious glial cells that abound in the brain. More recent experiments explore what happens at synapses within the brain when one nerve cell receives many thousands of discrete inputs.

Even Your Majesty's scientifically illiterate Public Orator in reading Professor Kuffler's Ferrier Lecture was able to keep going through a jungle of protoplasmic astrocytes, oligodendrocytes, glial cells and neurones, guided by an electron micrograph map of the cerebellum of a rat and a ganglion of a living leech, to reach at the end of the trek the conclusion that what goes on in the brain is an elaborate game of tennis. At least that seems to be one way of interpreting the author's statement:

> the basic observation is that if a nerve volley is set up in the non-myelinated axons of the optic nerve the glial cells are depolarized.

I request you, chancellor, by the authority of the Senate to admit Stephen Wilhelm Kuffler to the degree of Doctor of Science, *honoris causa.*

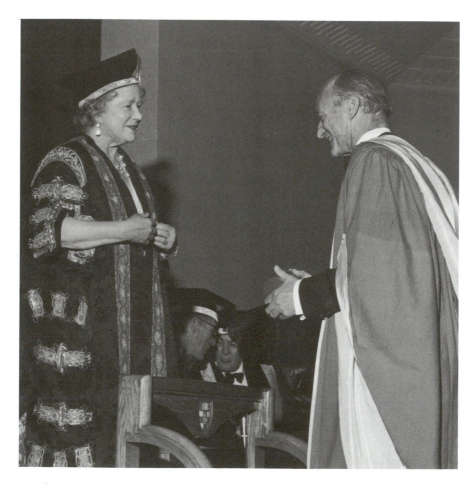

Steve receiving his honorary degree from the Queen Mother, 1974.

6

Carlton C. Hunt
Department of Neurology and Neurological Surgery
Washington University School of Medicine
St. Louis, Missouri

When I received a three-year NRC fellowship in neurology in 1948, I had planned to work in the Department of Medicine at Johns Hopkins. But A. M. Harvey, the chairman of that department, suggested that I might like to meet a young neurophysiologist, Stephen Kuffler, who had just arrived there from Australia via Chicago. He was setting up a lab in the basement of the Wilmer Institute. If it were agreeable to us both, Harvey thought I might like to spend my first year working with him. It proved agreeable indeed and we worked together for four years. I have always been grateful to Mac Harvey for providing me with the opportunity that changed the course of my life.

At first there was only Steve, Bob Bosler, and me in the lab. The problem we undertook was the function of the small-diameter ventral root axons to muscle in mammals. Steve's studies with Gerard, and with Laporte and Ransmeier, had shown that the motor axons of small diameter, in frog, innervated tonic extrafusal fibres, but there were still two views about their function in mammals. Most studies, particularly those of Leksell, suggested they were motor to muscle spindles, but Hagquist held that they innervated extrafusal fibres. After several frustrating months of trying to obtain a highly selective block of alpha axons while sparing conduction in the smaller axons, Steve had the idea of subdividing filaments of ventral root to obtain single gamma axons. It worked very well and we found that these fibres produced no detectable tension but increased the afferent discharge in muscle nerves, as Leksell had seen on stimulating the motor supply after most of the alpha axons had been blocked. I suggested we try isolating single sensory axons in dorsal root from spindles innervated by the isolated gamma axons. Steve was a bit skeptical but that too turned out to be fairly easy. We were on our way.

Our equipment was rather limited. We had stimulators, delay circuits, amplifiers, and a device for recording on film that sometimes jammed. To photograph the oscilloscope tube directly we would borrow a 35 mm camera from Mac Harvey. We lacked a mechanical apparatus for delivering controlled muscle stretch and because of that we missed several points where dynamic and static effects required discrimination. But we made a lot of progress in a field where little had been done and it was quite exciting.

Steve really enjoyed the in situ spindle experiments. We worked hard but had a tremendous amount of fun. He had a very quick and ironic sense of humor. There was much bantering and laughter during experiments which, when successful, lasted a long time. We lived in the same apartment complex and would sometimes race our cars home as dawn was breaking.

After I had been at Hopkins for about two years, Steve began to concentrate on experiments on the retina, while I continued working on the fusimotor system. I think he felt obliged to do something on the eye because he was in an ophthalmological institute. Sam Talbot designed for him what was called a triple beam ophthalmoscope, permitting visualization of the retina during introduction of a micro-electrode and the delivery of spots or annuli of light. These studies led to the discovery of the center-surround receptive fields of ganglion cells and provided the basis for the brilliant studies of Hubel and Wiesel who joined the lab soon thereafter.

This was a typical pattern for Steve. After a few years of work on a subject, he would leave it for his collaborators to investigate further while he moved on to another problem. He was a scientific explorer, leaving newly discovered areas to be settled by others. The number of areas of neurobiology he opened was amazing. But one field to which he returned repeatedly was the neuromuscular junction, an interest which began in Sydney. While Steve was highly respected for his many contributions, it is unfortunate that one well-deserved recognition was not granted.

He had many scientific problems in the back of his mind, often stemming from a chance observation or an old anatomical article. He did not operate on the basis of theory or formal hypothesis. He had a shrewd sense of where a promising biological problem was to be found, as well as a gift for finding the right preparation and devising an effective experimental approach. He was only as quantitative as necessary, but he had an amazing capacity of getting to the essentials of a problem. Working with Steve was a revelation to me, as it was for many. From him I learned how to design, carry out, and analyse experiments and how to think about biological problems. He was a master at dissection. He always liked working in the lab, and his publications represented work done with his own hands. His persistence and patience during experiments were exceptional. Writing papers with

Steve was also an education for me. One of us would write a draft and hand it to the other. This went on repeatedly until, finally, a mutually satisfactory version emerged.

Steve, a subtle, complex, and sometimes enigmatic person, had much warmth and concern for his colleagues, and especially for their children. He was very much at ease with children and his office at Harvard was filled with pictures of his large extended family.

Steve exerted a tremendous impact on modern neurobiology, not only through his research but through the people he trained and continued to influence. This volume bears witness to that.

In the years after our work together, Steve and I remained close friends. It was a bond which never diminished with time and I still miss him very much.

Carlos Eyzaguirre
Department of Physiology
The University of Utah School of Medicine
Salt Lake City, Utah

I was attracted to Steve Kuffler's laboratory for several reasons. Reading his earlier papers about the single nerve–muscle fiber preparation it was clear that he was an individual with extraordinary manual skills, possessing an unusual ability to design the right experiment to solve a difficult problem. He appeared to possess a Midas touch when dealing with research problems. This talent was evident when Hunt and Kuffler discovered the role of small myelinated motor fibers in modulating the spindle afferent discharge. This classic work brought the field of posture and movement control from the dark ages into the modern era. I was fortunate to be at Johns Hopkins at that time and had the opportunity to meet Steve. We became friends and I decided that working with him would be both a privilege and the best training for a young physiologist. This dream became true three years later when I obtained a Guggenheim Fellowship and Steve accepted me in his laboratory. I was on my way to becoming a sensory physiologist.

Two years working with Steve (1953–1955) on the crayfish stretch receptor were simply marvelous and afforded the opportunity to observe closely how this man worked and thought. His experimental approach was quite simple. Steve had a general idea of what he wanted to do. In this particular case it was to study the properties of the sensory receptor neuron. He planned the experiments a few days ahead of time, but there were no elaborate hypotheses (so much in vogue these days). It was like creating a sculpture from a piece of stone, sometimes following a sketch, but more often than not plans were changed as the work proceeded. It was an artist's conception without a completely preconceived plan. He insisted on having facts and the data well analyzed before going ahead with the next step. That approach, which proved so successful so many times, might not be too popular these days with peer review groups. It is easy to imagine their displeasure with an investigator presenting only a general plan and hoping to develop new ideas and techniques along the way.

Steve's sense of humor is legendary. There are countless stories in which his sharp wit was evident. It is unwise to repeat some of them since they could offend some people, especially out of context and too distant from the occasion that originated them. He had a devilish way of deflating egos and poking fun at famous people. Once we were visited by Sir Henry Dale, and Steve congratulated him on a recently delivered lecture, telling Sir Henry how pleased he was because the content of the lecture was true! This type of humor appeared during long hours of experimentation, helping a lot to relieve the tension and frustrations of the moment. As the junior partner during the experiments, I was always careful about what I said for fear of being hit between the eyes if my remarks were silly. However, this seldom happened even when justified, since Steve was basically a very kind and friendly person who took pains to make his fellows feel welcome both in the laboratory and at his home.

Wolfgang Trautwein
II Physiologisches Institut der Universität des Saarlandes
Homburg, Germany

Steve was my teacher and mentor ever since I went to his laboratory in the Wilmer Eye Institute in Baltimore in 1954. It was a great experience and challenge to work in his group. He created a marvelous atmosphere. His guidance was not by giving strict advice but rather by short remarks which after some thinking brought people onto the right track. I remember asking Steve several times for his opinion on two manuscripts which I had prepared in Heidelberg. His response was the question, "Why did you do all these experiments?" and the suggestion of some experiments which could perhaps solve the problem. It occurred to me that this was just the right criticism of a descriptive and rather dull work. This and other experiences, like the long, thorough discussions on the ongoing work after lunch in the mess hall, taught me the importance of choosing a really valuable problem and being careful when interpreting results. I only had the privilege to conduct experiments with Steve for a few weeks. His manual skill and patience in handling difficult dissections was an aesthetic pleasure. He also showed constant interest in my work with Otto Hutter on the sinus node, especially since he happened to mix up his film of inhibitory responses on the crayfish stretch receptor with ours on vagal inhibition. Except for the time scale they looked almost identical. Steve had exceptionally fine antennae for a good problem and the appropriate preparation to solve it. Slowly and systematically he developed a preparation and did extensive preliminary experiments before he began the experimental series proper. As a neurobiologist, he not only used electrophysiological techniques, but had a strong inclination to morphological techniques, and he was early to realize the importance of biochemical aspects.

Steve was an example in many respects. The vigor he showed in everything he did, especially in his experimental work, stimulated his coworkers very much, and his integrity and kind personality had many admirers. His profound and humanistic background struck me when he wrote an address of several pages in Latin (without a dictionary) on the occasion of an honorary degree given to him in Bern. I was very impressed, and Steve in his modest way said, "You know we had to talk Latin in the last three classes in the Kalksburg in Vienna" (a *Gymnasium* with a high reputation which still exists). After I had left the laboratory, Steve was my "extension teacher" until his death. I am indebted to him for his valuable criticism and much good advice. My wife and I had the privilege to be among his friends, and we had the pleasure of his visits to Heidelberg and Homburg as well as the very enjoyable days in Boston and Woods Hole. I shall never forget a summer vacation with Steve's family and the family of a Viennese friend and classmate of his at the lake of Millstadt in Austria. I never saw him laughing as much as this summer when the old school boys remembered their school pranks. I always felt that the time with Steve influenced me greatly and I owe him very much. With nostalgic feeling I remember this sensitive and kind teacher and friend.

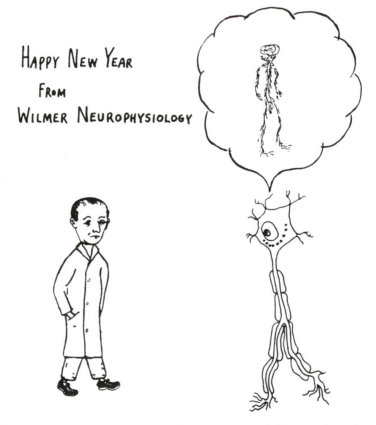

HAPPY NEW YEAR
FROM
WILMER NEUROPHYSIOLOGY

New Year's card sent by Steve to colleagues ca. 1950. He continued sending out yearly greetings until the early 1970s.

Josef Dudel
Physiologisches Institut der Technischen
Universität München
München, Germany

My beginnings in electrophysiology were in excitation and inhibition of cardial cells with Wolfgang Trautwein in Heidelberg. With his recommendation I had the luck in 1958, at the age of 28, to be accepted to the laboratory of Steve Kuffler in Baltimore, and to work on his team for two years. The program was to find whether GABA was really the inhibitory transmitter in crustacean muscle—which had been doubted by Ernst Florey—and whether the conductance increase of the muscle membrane was the complete explanation of inhibition. Fatt and Katz had indicated some quantitative inconsistencies in this mechanism of inhibition. In retrospect, these were central problems of neurobiology at that time. This is one example of the most impressive scientific merit of Steve Kuffler: He always directed his work and that of his collaborators to most original and central problems of neurobiology.

In order to tackle the problem of inhibitory transmission, Steve had formed a group of three neurophysiologists—himself, Dave Potter, and me—and two chemists, A. Kagi and R. Gryder (replaced in Boston by Ed Kravitz). The chemical approach was to homogenize the nervous systems of lobsters, to fractionalize all water-soluble substances in this system, and to test them for inhibitory or excitatory action at the neuromuscular junction of crayfish. This was quite a program at that time. Steve himself had no chemical background at all, but he had the insight that collaboration between neurophysiologists and chemists was necessary to solve the identification of the transmitter. So he got advice from friends in chemistry, managed to obtain grant support, hired chemists, and bought the necessary equipment. Steve did not have much academic standing at that time; he had just four laboratory rooms in the basement of the Wilmer Eye Clinic at Johns Hopkins Medical School. To start a long-range, multidisciplinary program under such conditions took a lot of courage. Steve did not take his responsibility for the project lightly; he was cautious in character and felt the obligation involved in spending a lot of research money heavily. Seeing the necessity of this project, and feeling able to carry it through, he made the big effort and finally managed. It helped that he was offered an Institute at Harvard in 1959, and that he could found there probably the first Department of Neurobiology.

All who met Steve knew him as a very friendly man, always helpful and full of jokes. He was very tolerant in his personal contacts, but he set high scientific standards. This is illustrated by the organization of the poor laboratory in the Wilmer Eye Clinic in 1958; in addition to his direct collaborators, only two further groups worked there. One was Ed Furshpan and Taro Furokawa, establishing the principles of transmission in the beautiful Mauthner neuron of the goldfish. The other group was Torsten Wiesel and Dave Hubel, who extended the concept of the receptive field to the visual areas of the cortex.

I have touched on some aspects of the career of Steve Kuffler which had great influence on my personal set of scientific values, and I am sure also on those of other colleagues. To finish, I want to report a humorous episode. In 1959, Steve Kuffler and I flew to the Friday Harbor Conference on Inhibition. I had to present, for the first time, the story of presynaptic inhibition in crayfish muscle. Most of the top people in neurophysiology were present at this conference, and I felt quite bad to give the talk with my clumsy English, having worked in neurophysiology just for a year. Medically educated and having taken notice of the existence of invertebrates quite recently, I was especially afraid of the zoologists. Steve encouraged me: "Don't worry, they will just ask what species of crayfish we worked on. And if you can reply, they will look astonished and say no more." This is exactly what happened.

Yves Laporte
Laboratoire de Neurophysiologie
College de France
Paris, France

I met Steve Kuffler for the first time in 1946 during a visit he made to Washington University. I was then working in Dr. George Bishop's laboratory, learning basic electrophysiological techniques from this generous and unconventional physiologist.

During that year, two French biologists, Alfred Fessard and Louis Bugnard, had visited many laboratories in the States. Their aim was to

14

find laboratories that would be willing to train young Frenchmen, especially in neurophysiology. They had asked Steve—at the time he was in Dr. Ralph Gerard's laboratory at the University of Chicago—if he would accept me for a short period before my return to France. Steve had agreed, and I worked with him in the summer of 1946.

I remember that period as one of the happiest in my scientific life, although the laboratory was not particularly well equipped and the heat was very trying. Doing research under Steve's guidance was most enjoyable: he had the gift to conceive "simple" experiments which worked, his sense of humor was sharp, and he was very friendly and helpful to the beginner I was.

The fact that I was so happy to work with him had an unexpected consequence. On the reprints Steve sent me over several decades he always wrote: "To Yves . . . à poil!" The origin of this odd inscription was that during the experiments we did together on the frog's small-nerve motor system, I often whistled a lively tune, and Steve sometimes joined me in whistling. A few days before my departure, he asked for the words of that song. I knew only those of the refrain; they were about "la première danseuse étoile" (the star dancer) who was "complètement à poil" (in French slang, stark naked). We had a good laugh, and since that time, "à poil" became something of a password between us.

Steve—everybody knows it—enjoyed making jokes. The one he made in Paris in 1949, during an international symposium on electrophysiology, was rather original and efficient. Steve's communication was scheduled for the beginning of the afternoon session of the last day of the symposium. We were all tired after a week-long meeting and not very alert when he started. It took some time, I am ashamed to say, before we realized that Steve was giving his talk in Spanish. Dr. Lorente de No and Steve had come from Spain, where Lorente had translated Steve's lectures so that he could give them in Spanish in Madrid. Steve, who had noticed that our attention needed to be raised, was reading one of these translations. We laughed and then listened.

It was also during that symposium that I saw Steve talking with Prof. Louis Lapicque, then a very old man, about neuromuscular transmission and endplate potentials. Today, the meeting of these two physiologists does not mean much for most neurophysiologists. For me, at that time, after all the damage caused to French neurophysiology by the isochronism theory of transmission between excitable cells (motor axons to muscle fibers as well as presynaptic axons to neurons) the meeting of the two men illustrated the contrast between the strength of well-observed physiological facts and the vanity of theories largely based on assumptions and a few uncertain observations.

Steve, whose manual skill was exceptional, always endeavored to develop experimental conditions in which precise observations could be made which were amenable to comparatively simple interpretations. This ability, together with a very imaginative and sharply critical mind, explains why he made so many important contributions in so many different fields. Undoubtedly, he has greatly contributed in shaping contemporary neuroscience not only by his own work but also by the many pupils who were influenced by his example.

THE BOYS

Hubel, Wiesel, Furshpan, and Potter moved with Steve from the Wilmer to Harvard Medical School in 1959. Kravitz joined them soon thereafter. From 1959 to 1966 the group operated as the Laboratory of Neurophysiology in the Department of Pharmacology, and then, after much difficulty with a conservative university administration and faculty, they formed, with Steve as its chairman, the first Department of Neurobiology in the country. Shortly after its birth, Hubel and Wiesel left the department to take positions in the Department of Physiology (Hubel was its chairman), and then just as shortly they both returned to the Department of Neurobiology. At the time of their return John Nicholls, a former student of Katz and later of Steve, and Zach Hall, a former student of Kravitz, accepted faculty positions in the Department. Steve affectionately referred to all of the founding faculty as "the boys." Also included as one of the boys was Bob Bosler, a senior research associate, who made the move from the Wilmer and was to become famous as the electronics wizard behind much of the group's success in electrophysiology.

All of Steve's faculty were at the very top of their areas of research and all were actively involved in teaching, but each was known among the students for at least one outstanding trait that helped make the department an exciting place in which to work. Kravitz's emotional good nature and interaction helped make the department seem like a family. Hubel was admired for his deductive abilities. Wiesel, who worked with Hubel and later shared a Nobel Prize with him, was a sober realist with apparently infinite patience, carefully analyzing all aspects of a problem before making a decision. Furshpan and Potter, who also worked together, gave the department a social conscience, which was of no small concern to students in the '60s and '70s; their efforts devoted to minority recruitment had a profound effect on Harvard and the field (as did their effort toward developing new and interesting ways of teaching cellular neurophysiology). Nicholls was the consummate lecturer whose style and method of preparation were much imitated by students in their attempts to master this difficult aspect of teaching and presenting research. Hall was the youngest of the boys and, thus, the closest in age and experience to the students; through him the students were able to observe how a junior faculty member goes about solving the problems involved in successfully establishing himself in his department and field while maintaining high standards. Nicholls and Hall left the department in the mid-1970s, but their influence persisted long after. Steve had chosen well.

Steve was as much a father figure to the boys as he was to the students. He led by working hard and doing excellent research, and by encouraging the best that the boys and the students had to offer. He was a master at avoiding confrontation. He used his gentle humor to let the steam out of things before there was an explosion. Then he would seek alternative solutions to problems that were satisfactory to everyone. His avoidance of confrontation served him well when the department consisted of only the boys and relatively few students, all of whom felt good will toward him. But as the numbers of faculty and students began to grow, this style became a handicap. There were too many problems that required decisions that would not please everyone, and the goodwill established over the years with the boys did not apply to the new arrivals. In 1973, when administration and the frustration that accompanied it began to cut too deeply into his research time, Steve turned the chairmanship over to Torsten Wiesel. He told me, "I agreed to be the chairman as long as it didn't require more than 50 percent of my time. Now it does." Steve was nearly 60 years old, and health problems were beginning to show. But he remained actively involved in the department's affairs, providing support and advice to Torsten when it was requested. Although Torsten put his own stamp on it, as did David Potter, who succeeded him, the department, as viewed from within as well as without, was partly Steve's until he died seven years later.

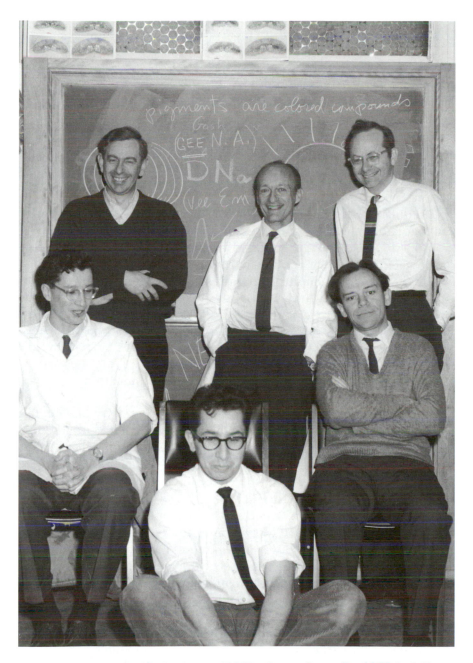

With the Boys ca. 1967. Back row: **Ed Furshpan**, Steve, **David Hubel**. Front row: **Dave Potter**, **Ed Kravitz**, **Torsten Wiesel**. Photograph by J. Gagliardi.

Robert B. Bosler
Woods Hole
Massachusetts

I first met Steve late in 1947 at Johns Hopkins Medical School. He had recently moved to Baltimore from the University of Chicago and was occupying a basement laboratory in the Wilmer Institute with the grandiose title "Physiological Optics and Neurology" stenciled on the door. I had just recently moved from the Bendix Corporation to the Department of Medicine where Sam Talbot, formerly of the Wilmer, was setting up a technical group known as the "Joint Electronics Shop" on the sixth floor of the Osler Building. I was hired to begin designing amplifiers, stimulators, filters, and oscilloscopes, also attempting to improve some existing equipment. Sam decided to temporarily loan me to Steve to assist him in setting up some electronics. The plan was for me to beat a hasty retreat back to the Osler to rejoin the growing technical group there as soon as the startup was finished. Fortunately, for me at least, that did not happen, and I went ahead helping Steve with the setup, using a vintage World War II Dumont single beam A.C. coupled oscilloscope, a Leica camera borrowed from McGee Harvey, an Offner amplifier, and a jury-rigged, jerry-built stimulator using thyratron gas tubes for pulse generators.

First, Steve got a collaborator from London, Peter Quilliam; a few months later Cuy Hunt, and then Gilbert Ling from Chicago, who had been with Ralph Gerard; then came Wolfgang Trautwein from Heidelberg, Otto Hutter from Glasgow, Miles Vaughn Williams from London, Carlos Eyzaguirre from Santiago, Werner Loewenstein, also from Santiago, Dick Fitzhugh from Hopkins, and David Ottoson from Stockholm. Then an even larger influx of people began arriving.

In the summer of 1950, Steve came to Woods Hole for several months. I joined him at the Marine Biological Laboratory the following summer when he set up electrical recording and stimulating preparations and taught in the Physiology course in Old Main. For the next six summers we would bring all the equipment in our cars, driving from Baltimore with roof racks piled high, trunks full, often scraping high spots in the road from overloaded springs. Those were the days before the Jersey Turnpike and Delaware River Bridge were built. Often there were many hours of delays at the ferryboat landings waiting to cross the Delaware into Jersey. Then through Jersey, then the Holland or

Lincoln Tunnel and straight across Manhattan, heading for the Merritt and Wilbur Cross Parkways, thence North to Providence, a city of interminable delays, especially since we could hardly avoid their evening rush hour traffic through miles of narrow, clogged streets. Then the final 75-mile spurt to Woods Hole, arriving often at nine or ten o'clock at night after spending 15 or more hours on the road with family, possessions, and equipment, all to be unloaded and readied for a summer of experiments.

Steve really loved Woods Hole. His final several years here were especially satisfying, since by then he did not have administrative responsibilities, and he was content to enjoy the pleasures of setting up preparations and dissections. On several occasions he mentioned that he considered himself very lucky to be able to continue working in the lab despite the cataract operations and failing eyesight. In retrospect, I consider the 33 years that I spent with Steve to be the most satisfying, productive, and agreeable in my lifetime.

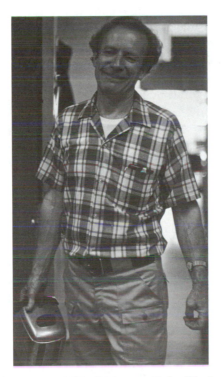

Bob Bosler ca. 1975. Photograph by Linda Yu.

David D. Potter
Department of Neurobiology
Harvard Medical School
Boston, Massachusetts

Steve was a remarkable personality, unique in my experience. Anecdotal memories of him are like fragments of glass from a stained-glass window.

Steve is famous for his willingness to help trainees, including inexperienced ones. I start with my own experience of this trait. I first met Steve when I took the Physiology course at the MBL in the summer of 1953, after my first year of graduate work. I remember the whole course with affection, but Steve's lectures on the small motor neurons of frogs and mammals were especially interesting to me; after the lecture part of the course ended I asked Steve if I could work in his laboratory for the remaining few weeks of the summer. Steve agreed. His kindness and that of his colleagues (especially Loewenstein, Eyzaguirre, and Bosler) and their collective enthusiasm made a strong impression. At the end of the summer, I asked Steve if I could return the following summer. He asked why I was interested in the nervous system. I blurted out that I wanted to understand consciousness; he smiled and said, "We all begin that way."

During the summer of 1954 Steve agreed to an attempt to record from neurosecretory cells with external electrodes, to see if the cells produced action potentials like real nerve cells; at that time neurosecretory cells had no standing in electrophysiology. Steve, Loewenstein, and Bosler were helpful and patient while I tried unsuccessfully to record from the eyestalk neurosecretory cells of the blue crab. At the end of the summer, I consulted with Ernst Scharrer, who was in Woods Hole. Scharrer recommended the remarkable pituitary stalk of the goosefish, *Lophius*, which in a large specimen is about 1 cm long, and assured me that the fibers in the stalk were neurosecretory axons innervating the posterior pituitary. Steve authorized a delay in packing the equipment for its return to Baltimore so that experiments could be done on a few goosefish. This kindness, and his help in sponsoring and preparing an abstract, struck me as unusually selfless behavior. I assumed that Steve would be an author of the abstract, as he had provided financial support, equipment, laboratory space, and frequent advice, but he refused because he had not participated

22

directly in the experiments. This, and a similar experience Furshpan and I had with Katz in 1958, made a lasting impression with regard to the significance of authorship and the obligations of senior people to trainees. I assume Steve was taken by the goosefish pituitary stalk; he is well known for his repeated use of unusual preparations to get at points difficult to investigate in mammals.

Throughout that summer and in my later years of association with Steve, I was treated by Steve and Phyllis as if I were a close relation. Personal warmth and modesty, informality, and an ability to communicate naturally with anyone, from babies to senior colleagues, were characteristic of him. My children called him Uncle Steve.

When I returned from London in the summer of 1958 to continue postdoctoral work in his lab in Baltimore, Steve asked me to join him, Dudel and two biochemists, Gryder and Kaji, in a new effort to identify the inhibitory transmitter at the crustacean neuromuscular junction. It was reasonably clear that the known mammalian transmitters, acetylcholine and the catecholamines, were not involved. GABA mimicked the transmitter, and if present would be an obvious candidate, but we were to extract and assay with an open mind. In some surprise I said that such a project might take five years. Steve said yes, it probably would. It took five years. Steve preferred such projects. That attitude is not encouraged by current funding practices.

During 1958–59 Steve was invited by Otto Krayer at Harvard Medical School to join Krayer's newly renovated and expanded pharmacology department; Steve was to head a laboratory of neurophysiology. Steve agreed to come if he could bring not only his own lab (including me) but also Hubel, Wiesel, and Furshpan, who were working on different projects. It is a measure of both people that Steve asked and Krayer agreed. Steve immediately recruited Kravitz to join this small group of electrophysiologists. Steve was an early advocate of the idea that progress improves if people with different expertise are stabilized in long-term collaborations.

By the summer of 1962, the GABA project was mainly in the energetic hands of Kravitz and colleagues. In his characteristic way, Steve was already scanning the horizon for a new project; I think that when visiting colleagues stopped expressing surprise or skepticism at what he was doing, he felt it was time to move on to something new. Glial electrophysiology attracted him; little was known and a lot was speculated. We spent a summer looking at the old histological literature in the MBL Library for promising preparations. We had a look at the dogfish retina and the nervous system of *Ascaris*, the pigworm, and finally hit on the leech central nervous system. The remarkable character of the glial cells in the nerve cord of the leech was confirmed, with electron microscopy, by Coggeshall and Fawcett. By 1964, it was clear that the leech glial cells do not participate in conventional moment-to-moment processing of information, and I returned to the GABA project.

This was my last direct collaboration with Steve, but like everyone else in his environment, I benefited from his presence in many ways. Two of his mentoring and administrative decisions that I remember warmly were that he did not admonish Furshpan and me for a prolonged excursion concerned with low resistance junctions in embryos and in cultured non-excitable cells, and that he supported Furshpan, Kravitz and me when we devoted time to minority admissions at Harvard Medical School. Steve's interest was new understandings, not conventional behavior; he exemplified the old Quaker prayer for the grace to accept light from wherever it comes.

Through Steve's persuasive efforts, and with the endorsement of an innovative Dean, the Department of Neurobiology was created in 1966. It was never Steve's ambition that the department should cover the waterfront. What mattered was an energetic, egalitarian, familial atmosphere that empowered a small number of innovative projects and collaborations. Trainees were honored. At the time of his death, he thought the department had become too big. He valued the earlier closeness and day-to-day contact with all his colleagues. He was freer than most scientists I have known of yearning for conventional rewards, and more concerned with matters that affect congenial productivity. I think that his contributions to neuroscience through fostering trainees and sound scientific structures were as important as his numerous scientific findings.

Edwin J. Furshpan
Department of Neurobiology
Harvard Medical School
Boston, Massachusetts

Although I never worked directly with Steve Kuffler on a research project, he was a significant factor in my life for 30 years. Most of the time I knew him was spent in Boston, but I think of him particularly in the context of Woods Hole and the Marine Biological Laboratory. I first encountered him there (in 1949 or 1950) when I was an undergraduate sitting in on one of his lectures to the famous Physiology course. These lectures, and the generally electrifying ambience of the place, were truly exciting. I believe they made my budding interest in physiology and neurophysiology irreversible.

It was also at Woods Hole, in Steve's lab at the MBL, that I first encountered David Potter, who had been given space by Steve to make electrical recordings from the pituitary stalk of the goosefish. Then, quite coincidentally, David and I ended up working together as postdoctoral fellows in Bernard Katz's Biophysics Department. Steve and Sir Bernard remained close friends from their time together, during the war, in John Eccles's lab in Canberra. (It was interesting to see Steve Kuffler and Bernard Katz interact. Together, they were quite capable of being silly—a word that was otherwise incongruous with Sir Bernard's demeanor and behavior.) On one of his visits to the Biophysics Department, Steve invited David and me to join him at the Wilmer Institute at Johns Hopkins.

Arriving in Steve's lab from London in 1958, David and I were soon enlisted in helping to teach in the Nerve–Muscle Program at the MBL. This was a summer course that Steve had invented some years earlier and, as might be expected, it was unconventional. David and I undertook to give some lectures and to help students with their laboratory work, but we suspected that the real agenda was elsewhere. The course gave Steve a chance to have friends and colleagues join him for collaborative projects (and good conversation), to find new preparations among the variety of local animals, and to infect young (and some older) people with his enthusiasm for working in the lab. Two of the memorable students in the later years of the course were Seymour Benzer (not yet at Caltech) and Ed Lennox (a senior immunologist at the Salk Institute), when both were testing the neurobiological waters.

25

Such students were, of course, enormously enlivening. The venue for the course, at the east end of Lillie, was a large open room for communal activities surrounded by six small rooms each meant for two students (or instructors) and an electrophysiological setup—an arrangement that survives, although in a different location, in the current MBL Neurobiology course. As with so many of Steve's inventions, it showed the way.

When Steve discovered, one summer at Woods Hole, that I also played on the clarinet, he insisted that we do duets—a stimulus for us to become more serious about learning the instrument. But, of course, seriousness was out of the question. Although we didn't invent the clarinet duo, we certainly gave it a bad name. There was no place in Woods Hole that was totally out of earshot of innocent people, so we were forced to take Steve's motor boat well offshore for our practice sessions. On some of these outings we forgot to take the clarinets. I recall one exhilarating trip back from Martha's Vineyard. It was overcast and drizzly, and the swells were impressive. The visibility was quite limited, but Steve opened the throttle wide and the boat flew and bounced, taking off from the top of one wave and banging against the next. Steve obviously loved it. He also wanted to share the fun and had me take the helm for part of the way back. Steve's capacity for enjoyment of things (small children, a new preparation, tennis, a new device, a pun, a new result, bad music) was marvelous. He may have been a private person in some ways, but his enthusiasms were always shared and were infectious.

After Steve was recruited to Harvard, accompanied by Hubel, Wiesel, Potter, and me, we inevitably became involved in teaching medical students. It was clear to David Potter and me that an earnest effort would be required before we could give a series of lectures in cellular neurobiology. For this purpose the peace and library facilities of the MBL were ideal. We spent a couple of weeks there before the course (in each of several years) reading, writing, and revising handouts and practicing lectures. Steve strongly supported this plan and arranged housing for us. I recall his turning up and taking us out to dinner (in his convertible, with the top down). I recently spoke with a colleague who had taken the Harvard course in the 1960s. He said that what he and his fellow students appreciated most about the course, and what he still remembers most clearly, was the daily coffee hour where faculty and students met informally after the day's work. He was particularly impressed with Steve's accessibility and friendliness, and

26

that Steve had learned many of the students' names—a contrast with other courses, and an important reassurance. He said that this experience still informs his ideas about what is important in education.

As I have been writing this, I have been aware of the irony that Steve would be at least amused, and perhaps bemused, by eulogy. But, then, he's only getting what he deserves.

Edward A. Kravitz
Department of Neurobiology
Harvard Medical School
Boston, Massachusetts

I first met Steve Kuffler via my good friend Roy Vagelos. Roy, who was then at NIH, was contacted by Steve and asked about joining him and four junior colleagues (Ed Furshpan, Dave Hubel, Torsten Wiesel, and Dave Potter) at their new base of operations, the Pharmacology Department at Harvard Medical School. Roy said he wasn't particularly interested in the nervous system, but suggested that someone in his laboratory (actually Earl Stadtman's laboratory, but Earl was on sabbatical in Germany) might be, since the someone (me) continually delivered journal seminars on the "brain." Steve and I met at NIH and arranged my first visit to Boston. In preparation, I reviewed published articles of Kuffler and Co., since my biochemical colleagues professed no knowledge of the group. What confronted me were papers full of incomprehensible squiggles, strange abbreviations, and gross cartoons (in the Kuffler papers). I'd never seen cartoons in journal articles before, and thought this highly irregular. In addition, my biochemical colleagues warned me to be wary, as neurophysiologists had it in for biochemists, ever since David Nachmansohn had "disproved their theories of chemical transmission."

My trip to Boston by train was uneventful, except for the start of a two-day blizzard. I arrived at HMS, armed with a checklist supplied by my biochemical colleagues, of conditions to be met for my potential appointment at Harvard. These included: a primary appointment as Assistant Professor of Biochemistry (certainly not Pharmacology); at least 1000 square feet of laboratory space and $25—50,000 in start-up money (well, things were cheaper in those days); and a starting salary of $20,000 (I think). Upon arrival, I was greeted by Dave Potter, who pumped my hand vigorously, strode energetically around the room, praised all us wonderful biochemists, and expounded on the brain, chemistry, the opportunities at Harvard, life, etc. My only memory of Ed Furshpan was that he was uncomfortable the entire short period of time we were together. Hubel and Wiesel eyed each other nervously as I talked about the biochemical basis of memory, and I don't recall anything of their perfunctory explanation of their work. Then came Steve. He heard me out, listened to my theories on teaching and science and my list of requirements, and then said something like, "Listen, you don't want to be Assistant Professor of Biochemistry, or of anything else, because then you'll have to teach. Space, you'll share with us. We'll make you a Research Fellow, and you'll see, soon you'll be an Instructor." He next offered me a salary only a shade smaller than my very small 1959 NIH postdoc stipend. "What we do have to offer you is a share in a really large Program Project Grant, and biochemistry will be an important part of that grant. You'll buy the equipment you need, and the only requirement is that you work on the nervous system." Now Steve knew that I didn't know much about the nervous system, and that if I had any sense at all, I would get involved in what they were doing, which was the GABA project. The amazing part of that visit was that I recognized immediately that Steve was right, and that this was the place for me. I couldn't really offer a satisfactory explanation of that realization to my biochemical colleagues, since my reaction was mostly an emotional one, but clearly what was being offered was the opportunity to prove whether I was capable of being an independent and, hopefully, a creative scientist. A little scary to a young, only 1.5 years post-Ph.D. investigator, but what an opportunity. Steve offered an environment peopled by hand-picked, enthusiastic, talented young investigators, whose research focused on cellular and systems neurophysiology, and he offered me (and Nico VanGelder, who was hired at the same time) the opportunity to be the biochemical part of that environment, *including* funding for my research, without any teaching or grant-writing responsibilities. I took the offer, but did arrange to adjust the salary up a bit.

I arrived in Boston just in time to see the cellular part of the group (Steve, Furshpan, Potter, and families) pack up to go to the MBL in Woods Hole, which left me feeling somewhat abandoned and unappreciated. Again Steve came through though, by inviting me to spend part of the summer at the MBL with them. My linkage with that institution actually began at that time, and this too, via Steve, has become a most important part of my life. It's impressive that even though I had a hard time keeping kids' fishing gear and bait out of my reagents, I remember that summer as truly productive for me, both personally and professionally. Moreover, the project I began working on, the attempted isolation of a physiologically active peptide from crustacean pericardial organs (we finally isolated that peptide only three years ago), was started ten years before anyone, other than endocrinologists, was interested in the role of peptides in the nervous system.

The GABA work began shortly after that, first with Dave Potter, who with Steve and other colleagues already had shown that GABA was found in the lobster central nervous system. Steve, Dave, and I were pursuing this line of investigation, despite the observations of Florey and Eccles showing that GABA was unlikely to be a transmitter compound either in invertebrate or in vertebrate nervous systems. Steve rejoined us in these studies when the somewhat daunting challenge was before us of dissecting meter lengths of single excitatory and inhibitory axons for analysis of their amino acid compositions by a rather unwieldy hanging-curtain electrophoretic apparatus. What I added to the project shortly after that monster dissection was a highly specific enzymic assay for GABA (from Jakoby and Scott at NIH), which made life much easier thereafter. One of the most instructive things about that period, other than the fun, fellowship, and excitement of the science, was writing up the results with Steve and Dave Potter. It took us months of writing and rewriting, and endless sessions of thrashing things out, to complete those papers. It was trying and ego-wrenching, but very worthwhile, and I try to recapture that experience with students and postdocs whenever we write a paper. The results, even in the high volume mega-paper world we now live in, were worth it. I often reread those old papers, still enjoy them, and they rekindle fond memories.

Steve treated us like family, and we were a family, with all the strengths and weaknesses of that fragile structure. I vividly remember a Sunday morning call from Steve: Kathryn—"Who is it?", me, whispering,—"Steve."—"What does he want?"—"I don't know." Steve—"How are the boys?" "What are we going to do today?" It was genuine, kind, and nice to be treated that way, and how different from the impersonal academic world that surrounded us. That personal touch was yet another aspect of life with Steve, and I certainly have tried to emulate it in the variety of programs, courses, and activities I've run through my career.

From Steve one found out that science can be fun as well as serious. A notorious punner, Steve also loved my jokes, and was my best audience and self-appointed agent. Occasionally he put me on the spot, like at the formal banquet at the end of a meeting in Norway. Steve was called on to make a speech following the meeting chairman and Jack Eccles. Instead he said, "Ed Kravitz will tell the suit joke," and sat down. I only had to start, "It's a story about Max . . . " and tears already were running down his cheeks. How could I miss?

It's funny, I've told these stories to many people over the years. This letter though somehow makes me feel that I finally am saying in public some things I've wanted to say for a long time about my very pleasant years with Steve.

David H. Hubel
Department of Neurobiology
Harvard Medical School
Boston, Massachusetts

I can't be absolutely certain how the term *neurobiology* originated, but I believe Steve Kuffler invented it when we had to think up a title for our department when it was founded in 1965. That he almost single-handedly invented the field of neurobiology, I think few would dispute. Up to the 1960s our field had everywhere been fragmented among different departments—anatomy, physiology, and biochemistry. He must have realized what an advantage it would be to get rid of such artificial barriers. He not only worked and contributed decisively in virtually every aspect of neurobiology; he also surrounded himself with a broad group who ultimately formed the department's nucleus.

I first heard of Steve when, as a Fellow at the Montreal Neurological Institute, I was asked by Herbert Jasper to give a talk on the visual system as my contribution to a seminar series. Knowing nothing about that subject, I went to the library, where I chanced on the 1952 Cold Spring Harbor volume, and found the two papers by Hartline and by Kuffler. These were fantastic revelations: in those days all one knew about the optic nerve fibers was that they responded when you illumi-

30

nated the retina. (My attempts to make head or tail of Granit's findings on color in the cat had been discouraging, to put it mildly.) When I was deciding whether to go to Hopkins as resident in Neurology, Jasper's comment was that with Kuffler and Mountcastle at Hopkins I could hardly miss.

I did get to meet Steve (and also Mountcastle) in the doctors' dining room at Hopkins, but was too shy to visit his lab. My chance came a few years later when, at Walter Reed, I started getting what I thought were interesting records from visual cortex, and brought them to Hopkins to show the head neurologist, Jack Magladery. He said that he didn't have a clue what the records meant, but that we should walk over to the Wilmer and show them to Steve—which we did. I can still hear Steve saying: "Isn't this *interesting*!" It was typical of him: if he was bored, he would be polite and vague. If he was excited, he showed it.

Luckily for me, when I was ready to leave Walter Reed in 1958, Ken Brown had just left the Wilmer, and Torsten Wiesel was without a co-worker. I had been invited to set up a lab in Vernon Mountcastle's group, in Physiology, but remodelling there was delaying things. Steve suggested I join Torsten for a year. The year turned into twenty-five! One evening nine months later I well remember Steve driving me home from Hopkins and asking me how firmly I was committed to staying there. That was the first I heard of the impending mass migration of all of Steve's lab to Harvard. I had been mystified by Torsten's insistence on our writing up our first paper quickly because we had so little time left. The fact that we all moved with Steve (Torsten and I were both demoted from Assistant Professor to "Associate") shows what a magnetic personality he had.

Steve was a wonderful mentor. Almost always cheerful, never sullen, a marvelous critic. For ten years Torsten and I gave him our papers to go over; they would come back with more of his handwriting than of our original text. We framed, and still have, his critique of our first abstract, and I can still hear Torsten saying ruefully, one morning on my arriving, "I don't think Steve thought much of our writing." Steve was also a consummate politician, gently having his way in apparently hopeless situations. To have a new department come into being at Harvard in the 1960s was the work of a genius.

I'm sure I do not need to expound on Steve's scientific style, his ability to invade a new field, open it up, make some stunning contribution, and, where most of us would have kept on turning the crank for decades, get out and repeat the performance in another area. It was just Torsten's and my great luck to be able to follow him in one of these areas.

I could fill a small volume with illustrations of his wit. I once told him I was discouraged by my failure to keep up with the literature. He laughed and replied: "You have to decide whether you want to be a producer or a consumer." Perhaps his most memorable line (probably a dozen other letters will quote it) was in a seminar in which he introduced Jack (not yet Sir John) Eccles: "He has often been wrong, but always about important things."

How lucky we were to know such a man!

Torsten N. Wiesel
Department of Neurobiology
The Rockefeller University
New York, New York

In the Spring of 1955 I had finished my M.D. at the Karolinska Institute in Stockholm and had taken one year off to learn some neurophysiology in the laboratory of Carl Gustaf Bernhard. One day I was called into my professor's office and was told that his friend Stephen Kuffler at Johns Hopkins Medical School had a postdoctoral position open in his laboratory. Bernhard asked if I would respond to the invitation to go to the United States for a couple of years. My project in Stockholm was to study the effects of various drugs on epileptic discharges in cats, and it was only of moderate interest to me. The possibility to do single-cell recordings on a different continent sounded exciting, so I decided on the spot and without hesitation to accept the invitation. I had no idea who this guy Kuffler was, but soon learned from friends and his papers. I started to worry about all my inadequacies, but by then it was too late to change plans. After a wonderful boat trip on a Dutch liner, I showed up that August in the basement of the Wilmer Institute.

No Kuffler was to be found. He was, of course, at the Marine Biological Laboratory in Woods Hole for the summer. Charles Edwards, another postdoctoral student in the laboratory, kindly helped me get my footing in this strange and foreign territory. I made a call to Woods Hole, and Kuffler kindly invited me to come for a visit, but I did not dare go, as my English was terrible and there was enough to cope with at Wilmer to make me sit still for a bit. The laboratory itself was sort of dingy and run down, but when Steve Kuffler arrived a couple of weeks later the place suddenly became full of life. He immediately realized that this Swede was a novice in research, and put me to work with Richard Fitzhugh and Ken Brown recording from single retinal ganglion cells in the cat.

Steve realized that I was lonely and invited me often to his home on weekends for outings and dinner with his family. I came to feel rather like an adopted son during these early years, and this feeling of Steve as a father is still very much alive. Steve had an engaging personality, and he was in the center of the lively interaction between neuroscientists and biophysicists at the Medical School and at the Homewood campus. Behind the quick-witted Steve I always felt an underlying sadness, which was well camouflaged. This sadness became more apparent first with the death of his close friend Joe Leventhal, a young professor in the Department of Medicine at Johns Hopkins, and then a year later when Jonas Friedenwald, a professor of ophthalmology at the Wilmer Institute, died. On our nightly walks near his home Steve voiced his sense of loss and a premonition of an early death.

In the laboratory, Ken Brown and I started to work on the intra-retinal ERG, a project Steve never thought much of, but he let us find out for ourselves. The following summer, while everybody was on vacation, I did an intracellular project recording from retinal ganglion cells, and suddenly Steve became interested; he later put an illustration of this work into his Harvey lecture. It pleased me and made me feel that perhaps not all my research was trivial. However, the real change in Steve's professional interest came when in 1958 David Hubel and I began our single-cell recordings in the cat visual cortex. He immediately realized the implications of our findings and was always very supportive. Steve had a custom of wandering into the laboratory for a friendly chat, during which he found out what was going on, and at times bored into us in a friendly but no-nonsense sort of way. Next door to our laboratory, Ed Furshpan and Taro Furokawa were carrying out their important study on the goldfish Mauthner cell. Across the hall, David Potter worked with Steve and two other colleagues on the role of GABA and other blocking agents at the lobster neuromuscular junction. Steve had decided to make an effort to develop research capability also in neurochemistry, and the Wilmer basement became the embryo for the Department of Neurobiology, which would be born a few years later at Harvard Medical School. The embryo was nearly aborted when Steve and his wife Phyllis had a serious car accident on their way to negotiate his move to Harvard. Their little Karmann-Ghia slammed at high speed into the back of a big Pontiac that had stopped unexpectedly. By a miracle both of them escaped without serious injuries; Steve was left with a visible scar on his forehead.

The accident brought us all closer and became symbolically the last obstacle to overcome before we all could be transferred to Boston and Harvard Medical School. Steve had invited Furshpan, Potter, Hubel, and me to come with him, and we all joined him with our families to invade the famous school. Furshpan and Potter came as postdoctoral fellows, but David and I were, to our chagrin, demoted from assistant professors to associate instructors. Steve's negotiating skills were nonetheless formidable; within a few years the Department of Neurobiology was born and we were all made professors. However, this was not a painless process, and the tough side of Steve came forward on

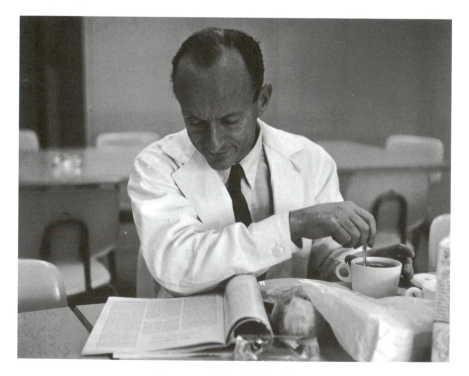

Photograph by Ed Kravitz.

occasion. At one point Steve believed that it would not be possible to obtain a tenure position for both members of the Hubel–Wiesel team. In my view he made the correct decision: he told me about the problem and advised me to look elsewhere for a position. Fortunately, before I made a final decision to return to the Karolinska Institute, the situation at Harvard changed, and David and I were able to continue our collaboration. During all this time, and until his untimely death, Steve and I remained close friends. I keep his portrait on my desk, and still expect that at any moment he may wander in for a chat with a cup of coffee in his hand and a wry smile on his face.

John G. Nicholls
Biocentrum
Basel, Switzerland

A charmed circle surrounded Steve in the early sixties. It was, I believe, Jack Diamond who recommended me to him and thereby let me in. From the first, as a student, I had found his experiments to have a unique personal stamp, style, imagination, flair, skill, and elegance. Again and again, important problems had been identified and plucked out of nowhere, and awful messes in the retina and muscle spindle had been sorted out. The style of the work is relatively easily described, the atmosphere in the laboratory and his personality are not.

Our experiments on neuroglia followed the remarkable opening that David Potter and Steve had made using the leech CNS. What I remember best is the talk. I tend to forget the hundreds of bad microelectrodes we made, the leaking of the perfusion taps, the horror of junction potentials arising at poorly chlorided ground electrodes, and the relentless search for stable, reliable glial resting potentials. But I do remember discussions about the "Anschluss," about Australia, electrical coupling, Jesuit teachers, and the dimensions of extracellular space. New projects were first tackled in an ill-defined, amorphous way, with no very clear goals, no restrictions—until somehow through experiments and discussions an idea suddenly yelled and took on a distinct form. As a teacher, he encouraged, planted (in secret) ideas for research that you later thought of as your own, and allowed you to do slowly and clumsily things he could do so much better himself. He

35

made my initial fear that I was not good enough to work with him (one I suspect shared by many colleagues) irrelevant: all I could do was my best. We loved working together.

The impetus for the book (Kuffler and Nicholls, *From Neuron to Brain*) was always somewhat unclear to me. I did not want to do it at all, but agreed because it meant we could continue to work together. We spent three weeks at the Salk working on the title. (I had learned from him that more than 99.99% of our readers would never get beyond the title of a book or a paper, so it had better be good.) And then several years were spent working on it only in the summers. We were well aware of its deficiencies; one year, in despair, we abandoned it entirely, only to come back later. The pleasure again was in the endless discussions. My main aim in redoing the book now is to keep his name on the cover.

I have not the art to describe his style, the wit that was sharp and quick but never caustic, the friendships that were deep, yet given to so many, the inventiveness, the feel for quantitative science without using numbers, and the generosity.

My favorite memory of Steve is sitting with him quietly in the evening once work was done, without talking, just friends.

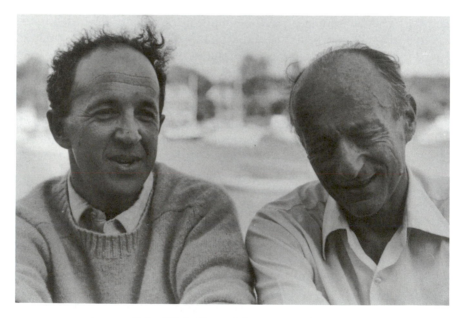

John Nicholls and Steve ca. 1975.

36

Zach W. Hall
Department of Physiology
University of California School of Medicine
San Francisco, California

In the summer of 1961, I was a student in the Physiology course at Woods Hole when I decided not to return to Emory Medical School, but to enter graduate school in preparation for a career in research. I did not know where to go or what to do. After medical school, biology seemed a luxurious feast, with too many choices. The only field that I could rule out with certainty was neurophysiology, whose Monday night seminars at the MBL I had found incomprehensible. In the last week of the summer, Ed Furshpan, whom I knew from the MBL dining hall, suggested that I might be interested in the group that Steven Kuffler was forming at Harvard Medical School. A meeting with Steve was hastily arranged—on the dock as I remember—and a subsequent one with Ed Kravitz, a biochemist from NIH who had recently joined the group. The meeting with Steve was largely ceremonial—brief, but cordial, with many smiles and few words. I had a long talk with Kravitz, whose ideas on membranes and proteins fascinated me, but I remained dubious that neurobiology (a term not yet in use) and I could contribute much to each other.

When I returned to Emory, I somehow came across a copy of Steve's Harvey Lecture, which I read and reread with wonder. It was my moment of epiphany in neurobiology. I found that it was absolutely possible to understand how electrical signalling worked, and more than that I was fascinated by it. I immediately wrote to Harvard and said I wanted to come. Thus marked the beginning of my involvement with Steve and with neurobiology, the two intertwined from the very beginning. What impressed me about the article was that it made such sense —a first lesson from Steve, who asked of things, both scientific and otherwise, that they meet the demands of common sense.

When I arrived in Boston the following year, I found Steve puzzling. He seemed less impressive than almost anyone else I met at Harvard, either in Cambridge or at the Medical School. He was not articulate, not hard-nosed, not aggressive, not outspoken. How did he ever get to Harvard? And where was the author of that wonderful article in all this? I tried to ask him "important questions" about his previous work, and was disappointed and baffled by his cheerful shrug and diffident non-answers. But as I hung around, the experiments kept coming: the demonstration of presynaptic inhibition with Dudel, the investigation of the role of glia with Potter and Nicholls, the early work on GABA with Kravitz and Potter. Each of those works clarifying, simplifying, leaving a field cleaner than it was before. In his turn, Steve was solicitous about me. Although he knew little biochemistry, he wandered by the lab and asked many questions about my work. He was also concerned about my financial situation. Did I have enough money? He once alluded obliquely to knowing what it was to be young and without money. Nothing as mundane as money should distract me from my work. Most of all he was interested in my young son, whom he always asked about with great enthusiasm. Genie, Damien, Julian, and Suzie, I knew from Woods Hole.

The pattern of our relationship, which continued until his death, was set in these early encounters. Steve taught not by words, but by example. His ideas were unobtrusive and uninsistent, but his wonderful experiments kept coming, and his work and approach to science were always there for anyone to see. He was always enthusiastic about my work and never failed to ask, not just what my lab was doing, but what experiments I was doing. And he always asked in great detail about my family. Talking about our children and our concerns as parents was a common thread of our conversations over the years.

Steve gave to me what he gave to a generation of young neurobiologists: the opportunity and support to do one's best, and a superb example to point the way. I still catch myself thinking—I will have to tell Steve about this result.

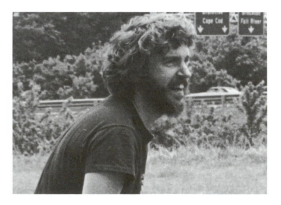

Zach Hall ca. 1973.

38

COMPARISONS

It is difficult to compare Steve with other biologists of his generation because of his breadth of interests and talents and his all-round success as an experimentalist, teacher, and leader. The following letters illustrate the problem.

Gunther S. Stent
Department of Molecular and Cell Biology
University of California
Berkeley, California

What is it about some scientists that makes people remember them long after their deaths? The all-time greats who changed our concept of the world of things—Galileo, Newton, Darwin, Planck, Einstein—are remembered as monumental statues. Others—Linnaeus, Maxwell, Pasteur, Boltzmann, Golgi—are remembered as eponyms of the principles, laws, or techniques they discovered. Most of the rest, if they did not sink into total oblivion, are remembered only as names in footnotes. Only a few are remembered as persons. It is not their outstanding scholarly contributions but their decisive influence on other scientists' lives that makes these few special. Stephen Kuffler was one of those few. Steve-the-Man will not be forgotten as long as any neurobiologist remains alive who came under his spell.

What was it about Steve that made him so memorable and gave him the power to dominate—maloré lui, it should be said—the neurobiology of the 1960s and 1970s? In my view it was not so much his undoubtedly landmark contributions to visual and cellular neurophysiology, or his undoubtedly fantastic intelligence, or his undoubtedly charming personality. Rather, it was his absolute incorruptibility, which set the highest standards of ethical conduct in a field which had long been rent by meretricious disputes. Without possessing temporal power, Steve had become an all-pervasive spiritual force, which drove the mountebanks from the neurobiological scene. He saved his disciples, who came to dominate the neurobiology of the 1980s, from falling into shabby practices: since having Steve think well of one's work was the highest recognition to which a neurobiologist could aspire, there would be no point in faking, stealing, or taking shortcuts. Steve would see through all dirty tricks.

I was especially sensitive to this source of Steve's influence, since by the time we met in the late 1960s I had long been associated with another man who also had this rare trait, namely Max Delbrück. By dint of his incorruptibility Delbrück set ethical and intellectual standards for the nascent molecular biology of the 1940s and 1950s that made this novel discipline very different from its cantankerous precursors, biochemistry and genetics.

As a freshly minted Ph.D. in Physical Chemistry, I went to Caltech as Delbrück's first postdoc. It was the summer of 1948. I wanted to join him in his quest for the physical basis of heredity, thinking it would provide more scientific romance than the statistical mechanics of polymers with which I had been wrestling as a graduate student. A few months after my arrival in Pasadena, however, I found out that Delbrück had lost interest in the problem of the gene. The discovery of the DNA double helix, marking the official birth of molecular biology, was then still four years in the future, but he felt that with the blossoming of phage and bacterial genetics, the problem of the gene was in good hands and would be solved before long. Delbrück had come to think that the nervous system still offered scope for romantic strife, and that its most promising point of purchase was the mechanism of sensory perception.

By the late 1960s, it was obvious that the fantastic success of molecular biology—the discovery of the structure, replication, and expression of the genetic material and the breaking of the genetic code—had turned it into the jejune discipline that Delbrück had foreseen twenty years before. Thus many of his first disciples, including me, belatedly followed his advice and quit the gene scene to take up work on the nervous system.

But how was I going to go about making this switch? My friends Werner Reichardt and Seymour Benzer advised me that there was only one way: Try to get into Steve Kuffler's department at Harvard Medical School. Seymour put in a good word for me with Steve—he assured him that I really wanted to become a neurobiologist and not merely to fool around with naive molecular biological experiments meant to show that DNA, or RNA, or protein, encodes memory. In view of the dire shortage of electrophysiological setups in his department, it seemed to border on irresponsibility for Steve to waste any of them on a total ignoramus like me. But, uncharacteristically softheaded, he agreed to take me on anyhow.

I arrived in Boston, in the fall of 1969, as a middle-aged postdoc, to take my orders as a neurobiologist. Steve suggested that I join John Nicholls, who was studying the leech nervous system. This very first piece of Steve's advice turned out to be the best counsel he ever gave me: I found John the perfect teacher, working with a nervous system that seemed like God's gift to a hacker like me with nonexistent surgical and electrophysiological skills. Now, another 21 years later, I'm still working with the leech. In fact, by now I've been a student of leeches as long as I had been a student of phages and bacteria.

Steve and Max Delbrück died within a few months of each other. The disciplines they dominated during crucial formative phases had come of age, hypertrophied from the esoteric research interests of tiny bands of zealots into workaday scientific mass movements. But Steve and Max had made neurobiology and molecular biology not merely nice places to visit but also good places to work during their *belle époques.*

Eric R. Kandel
Center for Neurobiology & Behavior
College of Physicians and Surgeons
Columbia University
New York, NY

I first encountered Steve Kuffler in the fall of 1955. I was a senior medical student at New York University School of Medicine, spending a six-month elective period doing neurophysiology with Harry Grundfest at the College of Physicians and Surgeons at Columbia University. Grundfest had graciously agreed to take me into his lab and suggested that I work with Dominick Purpura, with whom Grundfest was then collaborating on the properties of the apical dendrites of cortical neurons and their contribution to the electroencephalogram (EEG).

In 1936, Adrian had pointed out that the slow waves of the EEG, recorded from the surface of the cortex, could not be accounted for by the summation of fast electrical events that characterized the action potential of axons or cell bodies. More likely, he argued, the slow potentials were produced by other generators, perhaps by the dendrites. This idea was picked up in 1951 by H. T. Chang of Yale. Subsequently it was elaborated upon by George Bishop at Washington University in St. Louis. Following up on Adrian's idea, Chang and Bishop had done experiments which suggested that the apical dendrites of cortical neurons indeed had special properties that allowed them to produce slow and graded electrical signals.

Grundfest and Purpura took this idea one step further. They proposed that it was not the intrinsic electrical excitability of the dendrites that produce slow potentials but the summation of synaptic potentials upon the dendrites. By analogy to the endplate region at the neuromuscular synapse, Grundfest and Purpura argued that the apical dendrites were largely postsynaptic surface membranes and were therefore unlikely to contain a sufficient density of voltage-gated channels to be capable to spike-like responses. Grundfest and Purpura then tested this idea by examining how the EEG and other slow responses, evoked from the surface of the cortex, were affected by agents such as curare, thought to block synaptic transmission.

The questions and the experiments seemed exciting, but even in my naiveté I thought the methods indirect and unlikely to give clearly interpretable answers. Grundfest and Purpura, of course, were also concerned and talked occasionally about doing intracellular recordings from cortex, but they concluded this was not too likely to succeed.

It was in this frame of mind that I was introduced to Kuffler. One evening Grundfest threw into my lap the September 20, 1955 issue of the *Journal of General Physiology,* in which Carlos Eyzaguirre and Stephen W. Kuffler had published three papers on excitation and inhibition in the dendrites and soma of isolated sensory nerve cells of lobster and crayfish. Grundfest said something about Kuffler being very good, and that these papers provided direct evidence for the graded properties of dendrites, evidence that was consistent with what he and Purpura were seeing in cortex. I took the issue home and read the papers as best I could. Although I understood relatively little, several things stood out, nevertheless.

First, the figures were simply breathtaking; they were so clear and elegant. In my several months in the Grundfest lab I had read papers on dendrites by Grundfest, Purpura, Eccles, Chang, and Bishop, all of whom specialized in packing as much information as possible into a single figure. Kuffler's figures were different. They were simple, often making only one point. But the point was made in a way that was both convincing and aesthetically pleasing.

Second, Kuffler and Eyzaguirre were studying dendrites in a preparation in which they actually *saw* the dendrites and could record from them. For the study of sensory transduction they had utilized an invertebrate preparation whose sensory neurons resembled the muscle spindles of vertebrates. These sensory neurons sent their dendrites into the muscular element of the receptor organ, which possessed both motor and inhibitory innervation. The dendrites were excited by a passive switch of the receptor or by contraction of the receptor muscle. In the introduction to the three papers Eyzaguirre and Kuffler wrote:

> The greatest advantage of the present preparation lies in its accessibility, since all cellular components can be isolated and visually observed. Further, the state of excitability of the structures could be controlled and graded by utilizing the physiological mechanisms given by the stretch receptor nature of the preparation. . . . It seems of special interest that the sensory cell of crustacea possessed numerous anatomical features which bear a striking resemblance to many central nervous system cells of vertebrates.

Steve ended the introduction in what I later came to appreciate as a typically Kufflerian manner:

> It may be added at this stage that about two years ago when these studies were started, this receptor cell was thought to be relatively simple. As will be seen from the subsequent papers, the simplicity of organization of the stretch receptor structure is only a relative one and it is felt that many additional features of excitatory and inhibitory action have been missed.

This first encounter captured much of what I later came to appreciate in Steve as a scientist. There are always in his papers important questions. Then there is a wonderful preparation that seems tailored to address the question. Finally, the two are brought together in an aesthetically pleasing way—with clear, beautifully crafted illustrative figures. Still now as I write this I enjoy looking at these papers with Eyzaguirre and seeing how the stretch of crayfish muscle causes a graded depolarization that initiates a train of action potentials in the sensory neuron.

These figures summarized elegant experiments, and the experiments led to new insights. While I was at the NIH between 1957 and 1960, Alden Spencer and I often came back to these papers and their figures while studying cortical hippocampal neurons, now directly using intracellular electrodes. Here we encountered, to our surprise, fast prepotentials that we inferred reflected impulse activity from dendrites.

In a more general sense I learned from Kuffler's papers something about how science should be done—about the importance of matching a particular problem to a suitable preparation. Specifically, Kuffler taught me (as did Harry Grundfest in a different way) to respect the power of invertebrate neurobiology.

When I came to Harvard in 1960 as a resident in psychiatry, I had the opportunity to know Steve and to enjoy his friendship. Even though Steve as a person looms larger than any one of his contributions—much larger than the sum of his several parts—I often think of Steve's papers and I emphasize them in introducing graduate students to cellular neurobiology.

For example, I am much taken by the history of synaptic transmission, and particularly the "soup-spark" controversy. This was the dispute that persisted throughout the 1930s and 1940s between those favoring chemical transmission and those favoring electrical transmission. I have always enjoyed and encouraged students to read the important papers from this period spanning from the Eccles papers of the mid-1930s to the final remarkable review by Paul Fatt in 1953. One of the most striking and original papers in that sequence, and a centerpiece of any treatment of that controversy, is Kuffler's *Federation Proceedings* paper of 1947 entitled *Physiology of the Neuromuscular Junction: Electrical Aspects*. Here, Kuffler uses the single nerve–muscle synapse preparation he had developed (a single skeletal muscle fiber innervated by a single axon) to test whether electrical transmission can actually work as a neuromuscular junction. He asks, "Can the presynaptic action potential supply sufficient current to influence the postsynaptic cells?" He found that it simply does not, and therefore presynaptic current cannot be the mediating agent for synaptic transmission. He showed, for example, that subthreshold depolarization of the nerve terminals by applied current does not produce an endplate potential. Moreover, the prolongation of the depolarizing afterpotential of spikes in the terminals does not prolong endplate potential. From this Kuffler concluded that the action currents in the terminals are by themselves not effective in triggering the endplate potential; therefore transmitter release must occur. Kuffler ends the paper with another characteristically whimsical addendum. He has just received, he writes, a communication from Eccles, indicating that Eccles now thought that his electrical hypothesis can no longer be reconciled with more recent

44

experimental results on neuromuscular transmission. (By this, of course, Kuffler meant his own work.) Kuffler goes on to add that Eccles and his coworkers now believe the evidence favored acetylcholine as the sole mechanism. Kuffler was by no means alone in turning Eccles around. Katz—whose 1951 paper with Fatt provided the final proof—had been arguing this point since his 1939 book on *Electrical Excitation of Nerve*. Nevertheless I am told that Kuffler's experiments influenced Eccles greatly.

I find similarly inspiring Steve's earliest papers of the 1940s, written while he was essentially a postdoctoral fellow in Eccles's lab in Australia. Here, Kuffler introduced into neurophysiology (to the astonishment, I am told, of Katz and Eccles) the single–muscle fiber preparation that allowed him to study synaptic transmission on an elementary level. In the course of this work Kuffler repeated Langley's study of the 1920s, but now on a single fiber, and showed that acetylcholine chemosensitivity is restricted to the endplate in the innervated muscle fibers. Following denervation, there is a spread of ACh chemosensitivity along the whole length of the muscle fibers. I also like to return to the 1951 Cold Spring Harbor symposium on the neuron, where Kuffler outlined his beautiful experiments on the retina, describing the concentric receptive fields (the zones of inhibition surrounded by excitation and vice versa) that now bear his name. He also discusses here the relevance of this *opponents organization* for the integration of synaptic excitation and inhibition in the brain (there is much here that foreshadows things to come!)

Thinking about these papers conjures up Steve's scientific scope. We all have remarked (sometimes wistfully) how Steve never stayed with a problem but moved from one to the next—from the neuromuscular synapse to the retina, to the crayfish stretch receptor, to GABA and inhibitory chemical synaptic transmitters, to presynaptic inhibition, to glial cells, to microphysiology of the synapse, and finally to peptidergic transmission. In this recitation I am reminded of Isaiah Berlin's essay on Tolstoy, in which he divides thinkers into two groups: hedgehogs or foxes. The hedgehog knows one thing well; the fox knows many things. Most of us are hedgehogs (at best); Steve was a fox. He may, as far as neurobiology is concerned, prove to be the last of the great foxes.

Steve was at his best—his most creative—as a matchmaker. Steve complained that he tired of problems and hated to repeat even parts of the same material. ("Poor Bernard, he always has to give the same talk!") He liked best the *new* encounter—the search for the new preparation—that would best fit the *new* problem he was interested in. He then used the preparation to put his own, definitive stamp on the problem. Because Steve's approach was artistic and intuitive more than it was analytic, he often did not explain exactly what he was about. It therefore was possible to underestimate the depth of Steve's insight into a particular problem. Sometimes listening to Steve talk about neurobiology or about his own work was like listening to a painter speak about art. His description of science, particularly his own science, often did not approach in clarity what the work said for itself.

A remembrance of Steve as a scientist of great biological intuition who wrote elegant and important papers represents only one third of my picture of him. I mention the other two thirds only briefly. First, Steve made a permanent imprint in our field by founding the first neural science department. Steve, Furshpan, Potter, and Kravitz (the membrane boys), and Hubel and Wiesel (the brain boys), realized early that the various strands of the brain sciences—neurophysiology, pharmacology, anatomy, and biochemistry—needed to be brought together in a unified discipline. Much of what we now enjoy in neuroscience came from that realization. Steve infused the merger—the new science and the new teaching—with a high standard that endures. Moreover, Steve brought to neurobiology an exuberant, almost juvenile enjoyment of the scientific enterprise. One of the things most of us treasure most about Steve was his sense of what science should be. It was Steve's sense of neural science as a field for young people filled with excitement and fun that made him so inspiring to be around and made young scientists feel so welcome in his presence.

Finally, and most meaningfully in personal terms, Steve was a friend and counselor of immeasurable strength and generosity. Years after I left Harvard he would call on an occasional weekend to describe a paper he found interesting, or simply to inquire about Denise, Paul, Minouche or me. He took an intense interest in people, their careers, and their families. When he sent me a copy of his book with John Nicholls, he inscribed it, "This is meant for Paul and Minouche." (Our son was then 14, our daughter 10.) In writing this I sense how much he is still here. Next to Alden Spencer there is no other colleague in science that I have lost that I think of and miss more.

Yuh Nung Jan and Lily Yeh Jan
Department of Physiology
University of California School of Medicine
San Francisco, California

Between October 1977 and June 1979, we were postdoctoral fellows in Steve Kuffler's lab. The pathway that led us to Steve's lab was a bit of a roundabout way, and the experience was valuable and rewarding.

In 1968, we came from Taiwan to study theoretical physics at Caltech. After a couple of years, we became very interested in biology and switched to the biology division at Caltech in 1970. Luckily for us, Max Delbrück took us into his lab as beginning graduate students in spite of our total ignorance of biology. Max was a marvelous mentor and a remarkable person. We learned from him a great deal both about biology and about how to be a scientist; for instance, the importance of not doing fashionable science.

While in Max's lab, we gradually developed interests in neurobiology. We were very much attracted by Seymour Benzer's elegant work on *Drosophila*. Seymour has always been very picky in choosing people to join his lab. Initially, he was not very keen in having us. Fortunately, Max managed to persuade him to change his mind. The time we spent in Seymour's lab as postdocs was very enjoyable and intellectually stimulating. Seymour himself was great fun to be with. He attracted a somewhat eccentric but very talented group of people. Alain Ghysen, Chip Quinn, Ilan Deak, Yadin Dudai, Don Ready, Duncan Byers and Bill Harris were there the year we joined the group. Several of us were owls with respect to our circadian rhythm. Each day, around noontime, we staggered into Seymour's tiny lunchroom. We ate our lunch and had lively and free-flowing conversations on whatever subjects came to mind, which usually were a mixture of science, gossip, movies, and invariably, food. Such sessions often lasted well into the late afternoon. Serious work was done in the evenings. Seymour was good friends with many prominent scientists. Occasionally, one of them would join us in those lunches. That was how we first met Steve. Other vivid memories of the lunch guests include the great Caltech physicist Richard Feynman. One day he asked about what the group was doing with *Drosophila* learning, and in an afternoon, he managed to think of every clever experiment that had taken several of us months

47

to come up with. Fortunately for our egos, he did not think of new ones. Nevertheless, his mind was truly impressive.

At that time, *Drosophila* neurobiology was certainly not in the mainstream of either neurobiology or *Drosophila* biology. Moreover, Gunther Stent was writing articles and giving talks arguing that a genetic approach to problems in neurobiology (especially development) was doomed. Once in the mid-1970s, one of us gave a talk at a national *Drosophila* meeting. There were about 10 people in the audience. The neurobiology session at this year's *Drosophila* meeting drew over 300 people. A frightening mob scene. How times have changed.

The three years we spent in Seymour's lab were both enjoyable and very productive, scientifically and otherwise. One of the projects that we spent a lot of time with was the analysis of *Shaker* mutants. Based on the electrophysiological experiments we did in collaboration with Mike Dennis, we proposed that *Shaker* is likely to be a structural gene for a potassium channel. We even ventured the suggestion that by cloning *Shaker* one may get a molecular handle on potassium channels. However, at the time, cloning was in its infancy. We were certainly not prepared to take on such a task. So we were wondering what to do next. We asked Mike Dennis for advice. He thought that it might be a good idea for us to go to Harvard Medical School to work with Steve Kuffler. At that time, the Department of Neurobiology at HMS was *the* neurobiology department in the country. A lot of good people were there then. Spending some time there and gaining some hardcore neurophysiology experience could only benefit us in the long run. Seymour thought that was a good idea too. On the strength of the recommendations from Seymour and Mike, both Steve's good friends, Steve took us into his lab.

At that time, Steve was interested in slow synaptic potentials. Initially, he assigned us to work on the distribution of muscarinic receptors which give rise to the slow epsp. It was a good learning experience, but wasn't that interesting a problem. After six months, we discussed with Steve the possibility of working on a different project. Steve kept a piece of paper on which there was a list of projects that he thought were interesting. Among them, there was the mysterious late slow epsp, a nerve-evoked potential that lasts for several minutes, initially discovered by Nishi and Koketsu. Hardly anything was known about these potentials. We were attracted to that project, and Steve agreed that together, we would give it a try, even though it was a highly risky project.

48

To study this, we thought we should first identify the transmitter substance. By luck, we found it almost right off the bat. We started the work in May 1978, with a really simpleminded approach of dumping on our preparation all of the known transmitter substances and whatever else we could find on the shelf or in the refrigerator and seeing if any of those substances could mimic the late slow epsp. In Steve's fridge, he kept a box full of all kinds of peptides he collected when he visited the peptide labs of Wylie Vale and Jean Revier of the Salk Institute. Perhaps Steve got those peptides because at that time, among neurobiologists, there was already some suspicion that peptides may function as transmitters. To save time, we took random peptides, three at a time (why three? perhaps because in drama or opera, characters often come in groups of three, witches, Norns, Rhine-maidens, etc.), mixed them, and threw them on frog sympathetic ganglia. One such cocktail produced a moderately encouraging response. We then tested the components one by one. The one that produced a response turned out to have a label saying something about LHRH. We looked up LHRH and learned that it stood for luteinizing hormone releasing hormone, a peptide first discovered in hypothalamus. Initially, we were not sure whether we were on the right track, because the response produced by LHRH wasn't all that impressive. However, quite a bit of pharmacology had been done on LHRH. The Salk group and others had developed LHRH analogs which were very potent agonists or antagonists. When we put those analogs on and saw dramatic effects, we knew that an LHRH-like substance is a very likely candidate for the transmitter that mediates late slow epsp.

Within a month after we started, we got a good candidate, then it came time to go to Woods Hole. Steve kept a lab at Woods Hole during the summer months. He had already arranged that we would all go and do electrophysiological experiments. Because of the new finding, we ended up doing mostly radioimmunoassays at Woods Hole, in order to demonstrate that frog sympathetic ganglia indeed contain an LHRH-like substance. It was an interesting experience doing biochemistry there. Steve's lab had a great electrophysiological setup but no biochemical equipment to speak of. (There was no pH meter, balance, counter, etc.) We relied on the kindness of our neighbors to do those experiments. The three months at Woods Hole were wonderful. Steve was happiest when he was at Woods Hole. We spent a lot of time swimming and playing tennis and yet we managed to get a lot of experiments done. By the end of the summer when we all moved back to Boston, we had pretty much established that an LHRH-like peptide is the transmitter that mediates the late slow epsp.

In 1979, we left Steve's lab and joined the faculty at UCSF. Here, we continued to work primarily on peptides for a few more years and gradually started some work on *Drosophila* development in collaboration with Alain Ghysen and Christine Chaudiére, until, one day in 1982, we ran into Pat O'Farrell in the corridor. He was all excited about a new thing called P-element and he explained to us what it was. Immediately, we recognized that this was going to revolutionize *Drosophila* genetics and molecular biology and realized that it was a good time for us to return to *Drosophila* as our primary system.

Looking back, the time spent in Steve's lab greatly broadened our experience in neurobiology. In particular, we learned from Steve's style of finding suitable preparations to solve some of the basic problems in neurobiology.

We were very fortunate to have the opportunity of working with Max Delbrück, Seymour Benzer, and Steve Kuffler during our formative and impressionable years. They are in very different ways each a very unique and marvelous person. As we grow older ourselves, we appreciate more and more how remarkable it is for them to maintain childlike enthusiasm and to keep doing science at such a high level throughout their careers.

COMPASSION

The following letters document Steve's sensitive handling of the problems and personal concerns of others.

Hersch M. Gerschenfeld
Laboratoire de Neurobiologie
Ecole Normale Superieure
Paris, France

When one has had the privilege of knowing and working with Steve Kuffler, one may remember many facets of his personality as a man and as a scientist: the master of experimentation, the man who opened so many new pathways in neurobiology, the living example of original scientific thought. In this line I would like to remember his generosity as a friend.

I arrived at Steve's laboratory at a very sad and difficult moment of my life. A military dictatorship in Argentina was moving to destroy academic freedom and I was convinced that there was little chance that I would go back there. Steve had personal experience of such a situation and understood well my anxieties, and he tried to stimulate me to read, discuss, and experiment as the best therapy. His remedy was excellent. He passed me these messages during the experiments, crossing the barrier of my bad English by speaking a mixture of some Spanish (learned with Carlos Eyzaguirre at the time of the crayfish stretch receptor experiments), Latin, and French, all flavored by jokes and bad puns in different languages. From a year of work with him and Monroe Cohen there resulted a paper on the regulation of the K concentration in the brain extracellular space. When I read it again recently, it brought to me fond memories of our multilingual talks, and I realized that it is probably the best written of my papers, since Steve "corrected" (i.e., largely rewrote) it.

After my first year in the laboratory, he came from time to time to tell me that he had recommended me for a job or a professorship. I think that he did not much like my idea of moving to Paris. He wrote

51

a wonderful letter on my behalf to the French Research Council, but I know that he said to some mutual friends, "Hersch (or Hershie-bar as he liked to call me) likes big cities full of coffee shops."

I saw Steve for the last time in Vienna, where I had the luck of attending a meeting of the Austrian Physiological Society in his honor, that took place in a classroom of the old Medical School where he had been a student. He looked happy, and talked to me with nostalgia about the place. Probably the same deep nostalgia that I feel now writing about Steve, or when I look at his smiling picture in my office.

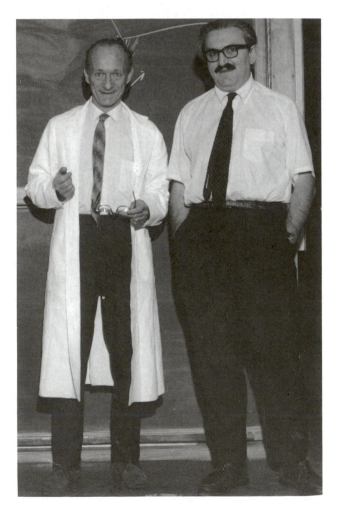

Steve with Hersch Gerschenfeld. Photograph by J. Gagliardi.

Rami Rahamimoff

Department of Physiology
The Hebrew University—Hadassah Medical School
Jerusalem, Israel

Between 1972 and 1974, Egil Alnaes and I worked in Steve Kuffler's laboratory. It was a wonderful period in my life. The atmosphere around Steve was one of intense work in relaxed surroundings. This is an atmosphere that I tried later to mimic in my own laboratory, probably not as successfully.

In October 1973, there was a dramatic change in my life. From our happy, joyful, and productive life in Boston, my family and I returned to Israel, three days after the start of the Yom Kippur war. There I was assigned to utilize my disused medical qualifications in a postoperative-care room. The amount of suffering that I managed to see was unbelievable. The person that helped me most to recover from this emotional trauma was Steve Kuffler. After the end of the war, I returned to Boston, this time alone, since we decided that it would be unwise to move our children twice during one school year. It was probably my good fortune that Phyllis Kuffler was at that time on a trip outside the U.S., because Steve and I had long walks and even longer lunches every weekend. The ability of Steve to listen was remarkable and so was his ability to put things in the right perspective. His sentence, "The price of survival is awful, but what is the alternative?" stayed with me for a long time.

Steve's sense of humor helped on very many occasions. On one of our walks in 1974, I commented that he was helping me a lot to get over my trauma and that he had very good qualifications as a psychiatrist. His instant response was, "I am glad that my training as a pathologist is useful."

After one departmental seminar, which was not very good, and which started with an elaborate discussion by the lecturer on his travel arrangements, Steve commented: "I think that at any given moment, about 25% of the scientists are up in the air," and after a brief pause, he added, "And if one takes into account also those that fly, the percentage is much larger."

Steve loved children and they reciprocated. It is amazing to see how, years after his death, my family still remembers Steve with great affection. But don't we all?

Marion S. Kozodoy
95 Leland Road
Chestnut Hill, Massachusetts

It was a lucky day for me in December of '66 when I received my first call from Stephen Kuffler! My interview was relaxed, friendly, humorous—with instant rapport. And so began a fourteen-year association as his secretary, administrative assistant, and friend.

Much has been and will be written about Steve Kuffler's scientific achievements. I can attest only to his human achievements—or perhaps I should say, his humane achievements. Over the Department of Neurobiology he presided like a father over his family. His colleagues, students, and staff—and their progeny—were all members of that family, all the beneficiaries of his caring warmth. To his graduate and postdoctoral students, each of whom had been chosen with great care and attention, he was always accessible for advice pertaining to their work, and to their personal lives as well. He took intense pleasure in seeing them move on to fulfilling careers, and to that end he was always eager to pass on to influential colleagues at Harvard and at other universities his enthusiasm for a member of his "family" of young scientists.

In other ways, too, he ran his department with instinctive tact and skill. From our work together I had firsthand knowledge of the regard in which he was held by the Medical School's administrative officers. Thanks to their esteem for him—and thanks also to his own unfailing ability to express himself in a concise, convincing manner, always with that famous touch of warmth and humor—he was invariably successful in extracting needed funds to benefit his department and its personnel.

Through his correspondence I was privileged to have a peek into many facets of Steve Kuffler's character. How many were the lives he touched, personally and professionally! His handwritten notes of congratulations, sympathy, or just cheery greetings were gems. Whenever his name was published in connection with an award he had received, letters would arrive from strangers desperately reaching out for advice to help their loved ones stricken with an incurable neurological disease. Busy as he was, he never failed to respond to these pleas, and often I detected a tremor in his voice as he dictated a reply explaining his inability to help.

54

Steve Kuffler's ready wit is known to all. He disdained pomposity, and was able always to dispel it with grace. One example is my favorite: during an honorary degree ceremony at the University of London, the honorees were presented to the Chancellor, the Queen Mother. Instead of giving the customary formal bow, Dr. Stephen Kuffler paused and inquired, "How is your grandson?" At that instant, he later told me, she ceased to be a queen and became instead a grandmother, replying, "Charlie's really a very nice boy."

Each time he returned from an awards ceremony and settled back into his office, it became my custom to inspect the wastebasket. This modest, unassuming man was prone to dispose of the program describing his accomplishments: he took pride in his work and in the work of his colleagues, but accolades and other tokens of worldly acclaim he did not consider important.

Stephen Kuffler enjoyed people, and in his presence no one ever felt uncomfortable. He liked to socialize—to be with "regular" people, not necessarily those who were his equals in intellect or influence. His spirits always soared when his own family came to the department to visit. I picture him now walking down the corridor with Julian slung on his back, or arm-in-arm with Damien, Suzanne or Genie. Children adored him. They considered him a playmate, for he was not averse to getting down to their level and playing on the ground. He was very special—he still is—to my granddaughter Emily. Some of her most cherished memories are of "Uncle Stevie" carrying her on his back through the woods near her home.

During the summers, in the unstructured atmosphere of Woods Hole, where he was happiest, the "boss" became again the concerned "father." It was mainly there that I was privileged to be a member of the immediate Kuffler family—ordered by him to relax in his lounge chair or told, "Go to the beach—that's an order!" The writing and editing of *From Neuron to Brain* with his coauthor John Nicholls provided an opportunity for me to spend prolonged periods in this relaxed situation. We were all working on the manuscript, to be sure, but my friendship during those times with Steve and Phyllis Kuffler and their children, and with John, is a highlight of my fond memories.

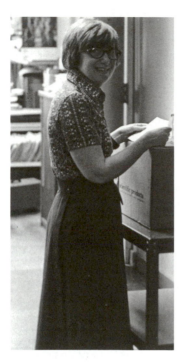

Marion Kozodoy.
Photograph by Linda Yu.

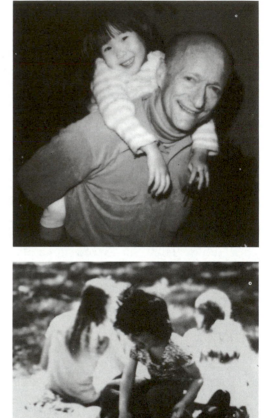

Steve with Marion's granddaughter.

"CAN MR. KUFFLER COME OUT TO PLAY?"

Steve was remarkably agile and strong. His extraordinary physical condition, until his last few years, no doubt helped him withstand the long hours in the lab. Once, very late at night after we had finished a long experiment together, I wondered aloud how many years it would be before my body could no longer take the beating. With a twinkle in his eyes, he quietly walked to a table, grabbed it by the edge so that he was suspended by only his arms, with his head facing the tabletop and his entire body extended parallel to the floor. Then he let go of the table's edge with one arm, and with the other he did two pushups, chin touching the tabletop each time. He was nearly 60 years old.

As noted above, Steve loved to play with children; with them he became a child himself. One beautiful Saturday afternoon in autumn I went to Steve's house in Newton to work on a manuscript. As I walked to the door I noticed a group of small neighborhood children playing in the fallen leaves, throwing heaps in the air and burying themselves in piles, all the while giggling and shouting with excitement. Shortly after Steve and I were seated in his dining room, where we were to write, the doorbell rang. Phyllis answered it to find the group of urchins shouting, "Can Mr. Kuffler come out to play?" He was out the door like a shot.

The following letters illustrate some other examples of Steve at play.

Monroe W. Cohen
Department of Physiology
McGill University
Montreal, PW, Canada

A letter from Stephen Kuffler to Joanna Cohen, daughter of Myrna and Monroe Cohen, five days after her birth.

THE SALK INSTITUTE
for
BIOLOGICAL STUDIES
24 June 1968

Miss Joanna Cohen
21 Wait Street, Apt 6
Roxbury, Mass, 02120

My Dear Joanna:

This is great! You are starting to bring up your parents quite correctly, timing your arrival at 2:40 A.M. Try to keep up the treatment for awhile and nothing can go wrong because in future, if you want to get up at 5:30 or perhaps even 6 A.M. they will feel that matters are improving greatly.

Of course, you have chosen very wisely in coming into this particular family, because from the looks of it, they are nuts about children. Apart from that, they are quite pliable—I wouldn't use the word plastic—and at a later date, you and I could get together to work out some appropriate strategy to keep the old folks happily subservient to your whims and wishes.

I have a few good ideas concerning your Dad whose weak points I have come to know quite well but I am less confident in your Mother and so I would advise you to observe her closely and make notes about her behavior patterns. There must be some crack in her armor somewhere.

I am eagerly looking forward to making your acquaintance when I return to Boston in September. In the meantime, give my best wishes to your Ma and Pa.

As ever.

Your obedient servant
(signed Stephen)
Stephen W. Kuffler

Jan K. S. Jansen
Institute of Physiology
University of Oslo
Oslo, Norway

As everyone who knew Steve will understand, he was the most popular of visitors in northern Europe. On one occasion we had decided to try late winter skiing in the Norwegian mountains. In late March 1972 we were on our way to a fairly isolated hut at the timberline some 400 km north of Oslo along with Anders Lundberg, Torsten Wiesel and Egil Alnaes. We were equipped as a decent Arctic expedition, and since the majority of the group was Scandinavian, fluids made up a substantial part of the provisions.

From the end of the road the supplies had to be sledged the last mile or so in heavy snow over to the cottage. In the effort, Steve, with slippery skis, unfortunately fell and broke one or two ribs. This reduced his operating range for a day or two, and he decided he should be in charge of the cooking and the kitchen. His only additional request was to be prewarned of any jokes or puns coming up so that he could adopt the appropriate position for his fractures.

In charge of the cooking, Steve soon found out that dried pike was the traditional dish of the region. Despite the fact that even the natives had hardly eaten it since the German occupation, Steve insisted that we should have pike for our first supper. After a visit to a neighboring trapper, then in his late 70s, he acquired a 20-lb pike (wet weight) of 1937 vintage and prepared a Babettian meal. By cooking in wine and with some juniper spicing, the otherwise rather bland-tasting fish was transformed into a savory treat. Linen on the table, warm plates, and pancakes for dessert, all prepared on the one available fireplace, established Steve's reputation as a "maitre de cuisine," and the "crazy American cooking pike" is still fondly remembered in the neighborhood.

Under the supervision of the medically qualified members of the company the broken ribs healed quickly. The most active part of the treatment took place in the sauna. This is originally a Finnish invention which has penetrated neighboring Scandinavian regions lacking showers and running water. The sauna strategy is to alternate hyper- with hypothermia, ad libitum. The photo illustrates the second stage—in the snow. Steve seemed to like it. In any case, the fractures healed without complications, post aut propter. The photo, albeit amateurish, is included for the benefit of other colleagues who might want to apply the procedure for fractures or other ailments. They should be encouraged by the second photo showing Steve on skis the day after the treatment was instituted. After a week or so we all returned to more civilized surroundings in the best of spirits. Steve even said he might consider repeating the expedition.

The memories of this trip, as well as those of all other associations with Steve, revive the rare experience of a warm personal friendship established at a rather late stage of our lives.

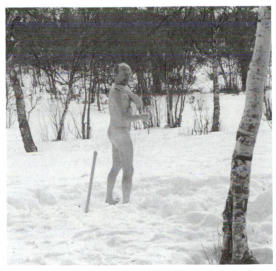

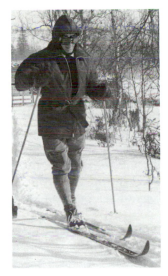

Steve in Norway.

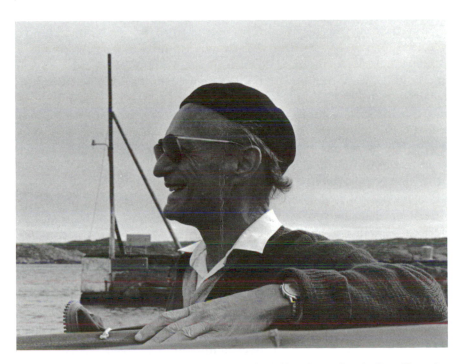

Steve in Sweden. Photograph by D. Hubel. (See letter by A. Lundberg.)

Anders Lundberg
Department of Physiology
University of Goteborg
Göteborg, Sweden

I first met Steve in 1949 through Yves Laporte, who had worked with him in Gerard's laboratory. He was not so much older but very much my senior in science, so I was full of respect, but he quickly broke the ice and we became and remained friends. He inspired confidence and was very interested in his fellow human beings and also in the "sociology of science." On several occasions he gave good advice regarding problems I had, both in New York and Stockholm. When visiting Baltimore, I stayed in his home, and I vividly remember being awakened by two or three children vigorously jumping on me.

During the '50s I only met Steve occasionally, but what a pleasure it was to be together with him at the Congress in Buenos Aires in 1959. Since then, we had many memorable encounters; the last was at the Congress in Budapest in 1980. Steve arranged a wonderful dinner in a garden, mixing his old Hungarian friends with scientific friends. We took half a day off from the Congress and walked the streets of Budapest. This was interesting since he had retained some Hungarian and could communicate with the people we met. On that occasion, we reminisced about pleasant common experiences; the foremost one was the visit to Bakkevolden, which Jan Jansen describes. Dried pike was not the only culinary experience—goat meat was another. We wondered why it was out of fashion nowadays and decided to try it, so we went to the old farmer and asked if we could buy a goat. He showed no surprise, but asked for what purpose. He still showed no surprise when he was told that we intended to roast the goat on an open fire. After reflection he replied that he would sell us a goat if we insisted, but would it not be more convenient to get a goat steak from his fridge? That was it, and the goat meat certainly matched the pike! On the streets of Budapest, we also remembered our mutual visits in Göteborg, and all the occasions when he joined me for a few days at my cottage in the archipelago, either alone or with Torsten Wiesel and/or David Hubel. The photo shows him in my boat. We went boating, swimming, and fishing, and we dined and wined well, but above all, we enjoyed each other's company, with Steve as the born leader.

When I last visited Boston my call was entirely social. He met me at the airport and we went directly to his beloved house in Woods Hole. He had no other guest and I was touched by all the care he took—at that time his health was failing. When we said goodbye in Budapest I told Steve that I wanted to visit him again in Boston. He smiled and said, "Don't wait too long." He knew he had not much time left.

OLD FRIENDS

When Steve felt that a colleague was serious about his or her work, he immediately set out to establish a friendship that could go on for decades. Some relationships were maintained by correspondence and an occasional get-together at conferences. Others involved more frequent and personal interactions. The following letters are from old friends who enjoyed a long-standing relationship with Steve.

Seymour Benzer
Division of Biology
California Institute of Technology
Pasadena, California

I first became aware of Steve Kuffler's existence in the 1940s when Lou Boyarsky, a former physics colleague who had switched to neuro-biology, took me to see Ralph Gerard's laboratory at the University of Chicago. It was a weekend, and no one was around, but I always remembered Boyarsky's mentioning that there was a terrific young neurophysiologist there named Steve Kuffler.

Not until 1959 did Steve and I meet, in a shop on the main street of Woods Hole, where I was a student in the embryology course. Steve was deep into the retina and I was deep into splitting the gene. As the conversation developed, we discovered something in common— Harvard. I had just declined a position there, but Steve had taken one. His move led, of course, to the founding of the Department of Neuro-biology, which was to become preeminent in the field and the source of neurobiologists now populating institutions all over the world (including five faculty members I later helped recruit to Caltech). After the summer, I returned to Purdue and the gene, having discovered in the embryology course that T. H. Morgan had done great work in embryology, but had thrown up his hands at understanding it and gone into genetics.

At Woods Hole again, in the summer of 1966, I became a student in the Neurophysiology course, of which Steve was the godfather, helped principally by Ed Furshpan, Ed Kravitz, and Dave Potter, with occasional visits by colleagues from their department. There were few lectures to speak of, certainly none by Steve, who did not especially like to hold forth; we mostly just pitched in and did experiments. Steve dazzled us with his skill at dissections for neurophysiological preparations. One memory from the course is that I persuaded a somewhat reluctant Ed Furshpan to try impaling one of the large *Drosophila* larval body wall muscles with a microelectrode. He applied a stimulus and the muscle twitched. Ed found that amusing, but essentially trivial, and was not interested in pursuing it. That preparation, in the hands of Lily and Yuh-Nung Jan, who, together with Bill Harris, got the idea years later in a Cold Spring Harbor summer course, led to a breakthrough in establishing *Drosophila* as a choice material for neurophysiological genetics. I suspect that the main purpose of the Woods Hole course may have been to try out prospective graduate students and associates for the Harvard department. This was borne out by the fact that, in August, Steve made a pilgrimage back to steamy Boston to consult with the Dean about offering me a job. I was tempted to accept on the spot, but another offer came from Caltech, where I was at the time on sabbatical to learn neurobiology in Roger Sperry's lab. I have always been amazed at Steve's courage in offering me a full professorship in neurobiology before I had done a single thing in the field.

Both Steve and I had been involved with the Salk Institute, which was then in a rather embryonic stage, but we both were reluctant to leave our established institutions for one whose future was uncertain. Ed Lennox, a fellow physics-to-biology dropout and a close friend of mine, had by then become a fellow at Salk, and came to visit Woods Hole that summer. He and "Furshpot," as the pair was often called, had done a neat study on the progressive closing of gap junctions in the squid embryo during its development. A camaraderie developed that highlighted the summer for all of us. Having three Eds around, we resorted to distinguishing them as Led, Fed and Ked. The climax of the summer was a fabulous paella combining all the species of sea creatures we could buy, catch, or steal from the lab. It was cooked under Led's leadership in Dave's house. So intense was Led's concentration on his art that, when asked to observe a beautiful sunset, he refused, replying, "By the stove, the sun never sets." Steve's contribution was, of course, a series of puns to fit every turn of the procedure. During that summer, my family and I had a cottage on the shore on Gardiner Road. On several occasions, while sitting out on the lawn, we were startled by two creatures emerging from the ocean—these were Steve and Torsten Wiesel, who had swum out from Stony Beach, quite some distance away.

All of us agreed that we should get together for scientific fun the following summer. But the question was—where? The respective advantages of Woods Hole and La Jolla were vehemently argued, with no evident consensus. So we resorted to a secret ballot. It turned out to be unanimous for La Jolla! The Salk was interested in maintaining some kind of tie with us, with the idea that someday neurobiology might become a significant part of its enterprise, as it has, in fact, now become. Under arrangements made by Led, we spent a series of happy Salk summers, Steve and I each bringing a few of our associates. As a result, I got to know quite well David Hubel, Torsten Wiesel, John Nicholls, and others who participated. Bob Bosler would drive a truck out a week earlier and arrange all the equipment, so that Steve could walk in and sit down at the physiology setup, his favorite place in the world to be.

One Salk summer, we decided to engage in a competition between three teams. The winning team would be the first to succeed in establishing neuromuscular synapses in tissue culture. Steve and Monroe Cohen chose the frog. They did indeed manage to repeat Ross Harrison's classic experiments, which brought them up to several decades earlier. Ed Lennox and I chose dissociated *Drosophila* gastrula cells and managed to repeat the observations of Robert Seecoff at the City of Hope, which brought us almost up to date. Furshpan and Potter decided on the mouse, but didn't get far that summer. The result was that, unlike the other two groups, Furshpot took the experiment back home and pursued it for many years thereafter, with many fruitful results.*

Among Steve's irrepressible puns were occasional aphorisms. He used to say, "*These* are the good old days." It sounded paradoxical at the time, but now, almost a quarter century later, it is obvious that he was right. The proof is in the photo.

*Seymour must have momentarily forgotten the beautiful and important experiments by Monroe Cohen and, in particular, the classic study Monroe did with John Anderson on the nerve-induced formation of acetylcholine receptor aggregates on cultured skeletal muscle fibers, all of which were the result of Monroe's initial experiments with Steve that summer.—ED.

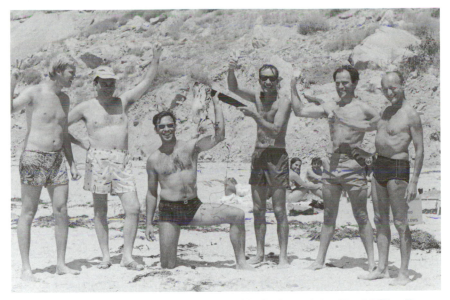

On Black's Beach at La Jolla, August 1970. Left to right: David Van Essen, Seymour Benzer, Klaus Peper, Bob Bosler, Torsten Wiesel, Steve. (In center background, Martha and Dotty Benzer.)

René Couteaux

Academie de Paris
Université Pierre et Marie Curie
Laboratoire de Cytologie
Paris, France

After my first meeting with Steve 40 years ago, I never had any but brief conversations with him, mostly during congresses and symposia. But once you were with him, you quickly realized that in addition to his gifts as a great scientist, he was, morally speaking, an exceptional figure, and although outwardly lighthearted, an extremely demanding humanist. And now, while I try to find words to describe him, I can imagine the ironic dissuasive smile with which, if he could see me, he would contemplate my efforts!

When I made Steve's acquaintance at a symposium in Paris, I was already familiar with his work on the isolated nerve–muscle junction,

67

but above all I was interested in his research on the frog's small-nerve motor system. This research, which Steve had started in R. W. Gerard's laboratory, in collaboration with Yves Laporte and R. E. Ransmeier, extended in vertebrates the work he had begun in Sidney with Bernard Katz, in John Eccles's laboratory, on the muscular innervation in Crustacea. The discovery of the small-nerve motor system enabled me to interpret satisfactorily some of my morphological and cytochemical observations on the different innervations of the frog's muscles, and marked the beginning of a correspondence with Steve that kept me informed about the results of his subsequent work with E. M. Vaughan Williams on the same subject.

In the course of our discussions about the small-nerve motor system and the "nice old endplate," I was able to grasp, very early on, the deep originality of Steve's views on neurobiology, which explain the impressive series of his discoveries, from his first research on muscle innervation in 1940 until the research that he conducted with such mastery on the frog's sympathetic ganglia right up to his death.

In this approach to the problems raised by the study of the nervous system, Steve always endeavored to combine all the data that could be provided by the most varied methods and was in this way actively engaged in preparing for the advent of modern neurobiology and its integration of the different neurosciences. For this integration to be successful, it was essential to choose favorable materials to which very different techniques could be applied, and this was one of Steve's constant concerns. Among all the materials he chose with his collaborators, many have become classic. I would mention as examples the ganglia of the leech for the study of neuroglial cell physiology, the crustacean stretch receptor neuron for research on presynaptic inhibition, and the extensor longus muscle of the fourth toe for the study of the slow muscles of the frog.

Another characteristic of Steve's work was the sober elegance of the style in which his articles were written. However, scientific periodicals give authors very little scope for initiative in the composition of their articles, and it was above all in the superb textbook he wrote with John Nicholls that his aesthetic wishes and preoccupations were best revealed. Nothing was left to chance in the conception and execution of this book, including the choice of the different types of print used and the minutest details concerning the illustrations. Steve was dreaming, as the Parnassian School of French poetry, of "enclosing the ideas within a perfect form."

The attention to form and the rigor that characterized the expression of Steve's scientific thought contrasted curiously with the continuous stream of jokes and puns that emanated from him, creating an atmosphere of gaiety in the midst of the most exacting research. His jokes were a natural antidote to the pompousness he so much detested. They were also in keeping with his indomitably independent spirit and acute sense of humor.

T. P. Feng
Shanghai Institute of Physiology
Chinese Academy of Sciences
Shanghai, China

Steve Kuffler and I had early common interests in the study of the neuromuscular junction. We first met in 1946 in New York at a symposium on neuromuscular transmission organized by David Nachmansohn. Then, following my return to China in 1947, my contact with the West was practically cut off for more than 30 years. In 1979 I got my first opportunity to visit the United States again, and I naturally made a special arrangement to go to Harvard to see Kuffler and the first Department of Neurobiology that I learned he had created there. On arriving in Boston, I was met by Kuffler at the railway station and we met again like old friends. I had a most interesting day in his department talking to various colleagues and seeing their experiments. Kuffler himself was then working on the late slow epsps in sympathetic ganglion cells mediated by LHRH. In the following year I was happy to meet Kuffler again and also his son Damien at the 1980 International Physiological Congress in Budapest. Soon afterwards I was deeply shocked by the sad news of his sudden death!

Although our personal contacts were limited to three brief meetings, Kuffler had left a lasting impression on my mind, and I have long admired his style of research characterized by keen biological insights, clarity of ideas, and neat experimentation. He remains a living influence with me and my synapse research group in the Shanghai Institute of Physiology; *From Neuron to Brain* and some of the original papers by Kuffler and his collaborators are required readings for young students coming to join my group.

W. Maxwell Cowan
Howard Hughes Medical Institute
Bethesda, Maryland

It is a pleasure to join so many of Steve Kuffler's colleagues and friends in sharing memories of the many ways in which he touched (and often changed) our lives.

Although I never had the privilege of working with Steve or being associated with the quite remarkable department he put together at Harvard, he was, with Le Gros Clark and Viktor Hamburger, one of the three men who most influenced my scientific career. For reasons I never understood and still find hard to believe, he took an almost fatherly interest in my work and never missed an opportunity to find something encouraging to say or to steer me in what always turned out to be a helpful direction. In the years I was at Washington University I got to know him quite well, as he was a frequent visitor to Cuy Hunt's department, and it was largely through his efforts that I was appointed first as a nonresident fellow of the Salk Institute and later as a resident professor. During my tenure as a nonresident fellow we saw a good deal of each other, and I have many warm memories of our visits to the various labs at the Salk and of our long walks along the beach at La Jolla.

As I recall our times together, it is difficult to select from all the memories that crowd into one's mind just a few that may be worth mentioning. However I think three stand out as being "typical Steve Kuffler."

One Sunday morning in 1979 I was awakened by a long-distance call from Woods Hole. It was Steve, who without preliminaries said, "I've been reading your paper on the isthmo-optic nucleus and I just wanted to say that I wish I had done that study." What praise could be higher, and could one conceive of a more graciously delivered compliment?

The second was at Cuy's home. Steve had given a lecture earlier that day and there was a dinner in his honor. Toward the end of the evening Steve seemed to have disappeared. I looked around for him but he was not to be seen with any of our senior faculty colleagues; instead I found him seated on the floor surrounded by a group of graduate students, not playing the scientific guru, but seriously listening to each student recount what he was working on. Steve always seemed to be most at home with the young and unpretentious.

70

And the third was when we first visited the Salk Institute together. Steve had not been there for about a year, and as we entered that lovely courtyard he saw one of the janitors on the far side of the court. With a loud "José!" he dashed across the courtyard and threw his arms around him as if he were greeting a long-lost brother. His total lack of pomposity and his genuine affection for everyone whom he regarded as a friend, regardless of status, was surely one of his most endearing qualities.

I shall never forget that fateful day when Torsten called me to say that Steve had died. It was as though a light had gone out in my world, and I knew, as I think we all did, that our lives would never be the same. It was not only that Steve had taught us how we should think about neurobiology, or how much fun doing science could be, but that we were among the most fortunate of our generation because we could claim him not only as our teacher and our colleague, but most importantly as our friend. He belongs forever to that select group of scholars who earned not only the respect of their colleagues but their deepest affection.

THE PIED PIPER

Each day Steve and the boys joined the students for lunch. Lunch was usually accompanied by a seminar followed by a lively discussion that could last well into the afternoon. The students participated in the discussions as much as the faculty and, following Steve's and the boys' lead, relentlessly probed for the essentials of the work being discussed so they could weigh its importance and make suggestions for improvement. Sometimes the lunchtime seminars were given by the department members. But usually they were presented by visitors from other universities who made a point of coming to the department, uninvited and unpaid, to benefit from having their work critically analyzed.

The department had numerous other devices to encourage this student–faculty interaction. For example, the mailboxes were purposely situated in such a small place that people literally had to bump into each other to get their parcels. Similarly, the kitchen attached to the seminar room was so small that at lunchtime it seemed occupied by a jumble of arms reaching for things in the refrigerator or on the stove.

In the early days of the department, when its faculty was limited to Steve, Hubel, Wiesel, Furshpan, Potter, and Kravitz, and there were few students, late Friday afternoons were devoted to a wine and cheese party, beginning in the seminar room and winding up with the group passing from lab to lab for a demonstration of recent findings. People from one lab would sit down at the setup in another and try to extend an experiment or check for a control. As the department grew, the Friday afternoon get-together became a beer party that included a mixture of scientific discussion and small talk that lasted well into the evening. To keep abreast of what was going on in each lab, the department instituted "evening meetings"; once each month the members of a lab gave a series of talks outlining the current state of their research.

The upshot of all of the interaction was that students and faculty came to know each other very well, the faculty treated the students as equals, and anyone could discuss his or her research with, and receive help from, nearly anyone else in the department.

The practical aspects of communicating to students how to select a problem, how to devise ways for solving it, how to weigh data, and how to write up the results varied from lab to lab. In Steve's lab, students were more or less apprentices. They worked with him on a project, watching to see how he did it. Steve never had a graduate student. I do not know whether this was because no one had ever asked, or because he had ruled it out. In any event, Steve's lab seemed best suited for postdoctoral students, especially those who had struggled by themselves as graduate students and came to recognize that they needed guidance. Steve was wonderful at encouraging the positive attributes the postdocs brought with them and, by example, he helped them overcome negative ones. Moreover, Steve was open about wanting to learn from his students.

The amount of interaction Steve had with students in the department varied from student to student, but none escaped his influence, as exemplified in the following letters. Spitzer, Rovainen, Van Essen, Frank, Shatz, Gilbert, Sargent, Stuart, and Nurse were graduate students; Patterson, Purves, Hildebrand, Muller, and Berg were postdoctoral students. All studied with one of the boys. Frank, Stuart, Patterson, and Hildebrand went on to become faculty members in the department. Cohen, Dennis, Hartzell, Roper, Yoshikami, and Horn were postdoctoral students with Steve.

Nicholas C. Spitzer
Department of Biology
University of California, San Diego
La Jolla, California

Steve Kuffler had a great influence on my development as a scientist. As a medical student at Harvard in the mid-1960s, I became very interested in extending my interest in neurophysiology. I remember my high hopes as I gave Steve my undergraduate thesis to read when he and others were considering the wisdom of taking me on as a graduate student. I was delighted to be accepted, and Dave Potter became my advisor. I started out as the first graduate student in the new Neurobiology Department.

In the three years of my predoctoral training, and one year as a postdoctoral fellow with Jack McMahan in the department, I saw a lot of Steve, as everyone did. I recall two interactions that stick with me most vividly, that seem to be quintessentially representative of this remarkable man. The first was an occasion, late one evening, when he had finally finished up an experiment, and came down the corridor in his overcoat, with his briefcase. He stopped into the lab, where I was busily engaged in experiments on electrical coupling in various epithelia. I am unable to reconstruct the conversation, but it somehow turned to values in science, and I remember with extraordinary clarity his admonition not to take any wooden nickels. He meant of course that one should adhere to the highest standards and be unflinching in doing the right experiment to answer the question, as he demonstrated by example throughout his career.

The second occasion must have occurred at lunch—then as now an informal affair, with whomever showed up. Somehow the discussion turned to the difficulties of staying abreast of a burgeoning literature. I believe that it was Steve who commented to the effect that in our business one may be either a producer or a consumer. I do not recall any further amplification of this remark, but it was clear where he placed his own emphasis.

Steve led a department from which quite a cadre of scientists set forth. Among the things that we hold in common, we are producers who take no wooden nickels.

Carl Rovainen
Department of Cell Biology and Physiology
Washington University School of Medicine
St. Louis, Missouri

Steve Kuffler said that you don't have to write everything that you know. In this tradition I shall be brief.

In 1964, Steve and John Nicholls sought a vertebrate counterpart to the leech preparation of neurons and glia. That summer at Woods Hole they made the first unpublished intracellular recordings from large Müller neurons in the lamprey brain, but because they could not record also from glial cells, they asked me, as a graduate student in need of a project, whether I would like to continue the recordings from the large nerve cells. Steve, John, and the other "boys," for the gift of my career, thank you very much!

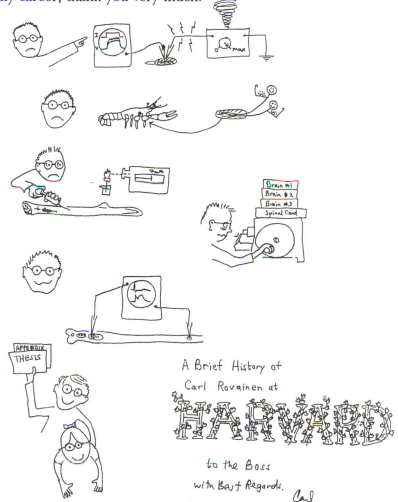

A Brief History of Carl Rovainen at HARVARD

to the Boss
with Best Regards.
Carl

David C. Van Essen
California Institute of Technology
Pasadena, California

When I pause to reflect on Steve Kuffler, a rich collection of images and recollections come to mind. Steve had a deep and lasting effect on my professional career, as he did on many others. My first memory is that of Steve interviewing me for admission to graduate school in 1967. This interview took place in the unlikely location of a waiting lounge at the Los Angeles airport, where Steve was waiting for a flight connection and I had driven out from Pasadena. Although the specifics of the interview are now hazy, it evidently went well enough, as I subsequently joined Eric Frank and Jim Hudspeth as the first official entering class (although Nick Spitzer preceded us by a year) of the newly established Neurobiology Department at Harvard.

The department was quite small at that time, and to a young graduate student it seemed in many respects a family affair, with Steve as the paternal figure. Of the many things that impressed me during that period, perhaps none was more significant than the general approach to analyzing scientific issues in a critical, hard-nosed, but good-natured fashion. This style was often evident during the many seminars provided by visiting scientists and by people in the department. These sessions were often highlighted by Steve's persistent, penetrating, but always friendly interrogation and his determination to pursue a line of questioning relentlessly until he was satisfied.

As it happens, these comments have been formulated during a return visit to Jan Jansen's holiday cottage in beautiful northern Norway, which was the site of a memorable winter ski expedition involving Steve along with Jan, Torsten Wiesel, and others a couple of decades ago. One of the highlights of that trip was captured by Jan's camera and is related in his contribution to this collection. I have often heard the story of Steve's hard luck in cracking a rib early on in the trip; he thereupon appointed himself as full-time chef for the expedition and became quite successful on the culinary front. This tale struck me as characteristic of Steve's resourcefulness, adaptiveness, and good humor in dealing with a difficult situation.

It was a source of amusement for many of us that Steve often had a notable difficulty in remembering the names of even those whom he saw on a daily basis. This frailty was more than compensated by Steve's genuine warmth, graciousness, and evenhandedness in dealing with people at all levels. He was truly a neurobiologist for all seasons, and our community was tremendously enriched by his numerous and diverse contributions to the field.

Eric Frank
Department of Neurobiology, Anatomy, and Cell Science
University of Pittsburgh School of Medicine
Pittsburgh, Pennsylvania

Of my eleven years' association with Steve and his department as graduate student, postdoc, and faculty member, three incidents stand out as illustrative of his scientific and personal approaches to life.

Even before arriving in his department, I was struck by Steve's warm, enthusiastic style. At the bottom of the formal letter of my acceptance as a graduate student, Steve had scrawled the line, "This promises to be great!"

Steve's intuitive feel for the importance of the unexpected observation was a hallmark of his experimental approach. While waiting the requisite month between submission of my written thesis and the examination, I got involved in the early stages of the ACh sensitivity mapping experiments with Steve and Doju Yoshikami. My full attention was focused on the positioning of two ACh pipettes, two extracellular recording pipettes, and one intracellular electrode (a configuration that, fortunately, was later abandoned). One of the ACh pipettes had been fortuitously placed right at the edge of the nerve terminal (this was before the days of removing it with collagenase) and the time course of the resulting ACh potential was nearly as fast as that of a spontaneous mepp that happened to appear on the same oscilloscope trace. This immediately caught Steve's eye. He seemed to lose interest in the sensitivity measurements, and I felt frustrated at his lack of concern for the experiment at hand. Of course, Steve had realized in an instant that the similarity in time courses meant that the ACh pipette was positioned right in the synaptic cleft, so we could measure the true sensitivity of the postsynaptic membrane for the first time.

Shortly before his death, Steve asked about my future plans and immediately offered this advice: "Try to arrange your life so you are doing the things you enjoy doing *now*—don't put them off to some distant time in the future." At the time, this variant of his "These are the good old days" philosophy struck me as irresponsible. Nevertheless, it has successfully guided my thinking on several important occasions. And the irresponsibility never caught up with Steve!

Carla J. Shatz
Department of Neurobiology
Stanford University
Stanford, California

My most enduring image of Steve Kuffler is dreamlike: a recurrent picture where the setting and characters are so familiar that it is difficult to decide whether it is fantasy or reality. We are all sitting at one of the several long tables in the Department of Neurobiology lunchroom at Harvard, at the beginning of a noontime seminar, munching away at our favorite lunches. In those days I always ate something terrible like salami and cheese melted onto a piece of pita bread (my concession to "health food"); Bruce Wallace is present with two or three peanut butter and jelly sandwiches, and Torsten Wiesel has his bowl full of special patented granola mix with yogurt, making all of us feel guilty. I can't recall what Steve has for lunch, since my attention is riveted on his face, which is filled with impish humor and is beginning to move. We all know that Steve is about to introduce the seminar speaker. This is the highlight of the seminar, since the introduction is always a combination of accolades for the speaker, plus jokes and puns, hilarious and often painful. This is why we are here; the seminar is only secondary. I had always hoped that someday I would return, grown up, to the Department of Neurobiology, and have the honor and torture of being introduced by Steve. Sadly, he died before this secret wish could be granted.

When I was a graduate student with David Hubel and Torsten Wiesel, Steve Kuffler was chairman of the department, with his office located just about as far away from my little space as could be. The department was in Building B at Harvard Medical School, with a U-shaped floor plan. Hubel and Wiesel had their empire along one side of the U, along with John Nicholls and Zach Hall, while Steve,

78

Furshpan, Potter and Kravitz were located on the other side. The base of the U was common territory: the seminar/lunchroom, the library, and Steve's office and lab. The physical configuration, and my own scientific interests, minimized my daily interactions with Steve; to me during those years he was essentially a benevolent dictator. It is only now, in thinking about my relationship to him, that I realize that without him, I would not be here as an active scientist today.

I believe that scientific relationships are like personal ones, but frequently they are more intense. After all, how often do we spend eight to ten hours, day after day, with our loved ones at home? I have long thought of Hubel and Wiesel as my scientific parents (don't ask who is mom and who is dad—I have no idea), and my cohort student colleagues as my siblings, younger and older. I remember with great appreciation and fondness the environment that Hubel and Wiesel created for us kids—the support, the friendships. Many of us literally lived in the department, cooking elaborate dinners in the small kitchen, consuming tons of cookies at teatime, playing soccer on Friday afternoons. This family atmosphere existed because of Steve's encouragement, patronage, and vision. It was Steve who catalyzed the collaboration between Hubel and Wiesel when they were at Johns Hopkins University, it was Steve who brought them to Harvard when he became chairman, and so it was Steve who made it possible for me to become a child of the Department of Neurobiology. Although I could not know Steve Kuffler well on a personal level, he is my scientific grandfather, and great-grandfather to my own students. He has created a lineage of neurobiologists who, I hope, will continue to make contributions that live up to his own high standards of science and personal conduct.

Charles Gilbert
Department of Neurobiology
The Rockefeller University
New York, New York

For me, Steve set the tone for the style and attitude towards how one approaches science. I got to know Steve from the time that I arrived at Harvard Neurobiology as a student. He seemed at the same time an easygoing and jocular, yet extremely hardworking scientist. He was very informal, and it was easy for students to talk to him on a first-name basis. He made it seem entirely natural for science to be done, even at the age of 60 or so years, with one's own hands, in collaboration with at most two other people. He brought a clarity to how one thinks about a problem, and this was reflected in the character of intellectual interchange in lunch seminars, journal clubs, and evening meetings. This led to an eagerness on the part of many people in the department to pin a seminar speaker down, to really get to the nub of a problem, and to evaluate the validity of the evidence. For people visiting from outside the department, this was often taken as harsh criticism. People were not allowed even the luxury of euphemisms in their speech. If someone said, in their description of their procedures, that they "sacrificed" an animal, Steve would invariably ask if the ceremony involved the burning of incense.

These days the environment of science seems very different from what I had come to expect from my days as a fledgling neurobiologist. One frequently encounters research that muddies the waters rather than providing compelling new ideas, scientists who operate large empires as administrators rather than working a single problem with their own hands, a star system honoring those having a few isolated findings rather than rewarding those who carefully and systematically develop a theme over a period of time. Steve managed to make major strides with modest resources. It's hard to give up the idea that Steve's contributions to science will be the most lasting, and that his approach was the most genuine.

It was always clear with Steve that the *raison d'etre* of a scientist's existence was to discover something new. Anything else seemed frivolous. He clearly admired most those students and postdocs who worked the longest hours. Science was a hands-on activity. If someone received a high starting salary at another institution, it seemed to Steve that the person had questionable motives. In most things Steve strove for a simple, unadorned lifestyle, sometimes bordering on a Spartan existence. When I traveled with Torsten and Steve through Italy after attending a meeting in Rome, in every Italian restaurant, despite the tempting variety of things on the menu, time after time Steve ordered Wiener schnitzel, or the Italian equivalent. Finally after several days of this, Torsten insisted that Steve order something else. On this trip Steve's diabetes was a real problem, it was not very well managed, but even so he would insist on going on every hike, on climbing yet another peak.

Steve's approach towards science turned out to be rarer than I expected, but it helps one separate the authentic work from the dross.

Peter B. Sargent

**Departments of Stomatology and Physiology and the Neuroscience Graduate Program
University of California
San Francisco, California**

Sometime in the winter of 1975–76, Steve visited UCSF, where I was a postdoctoral fellow with Mike Dennis in the Department of Physiology. During that visit I sat down with Steve to tell him about some new results Mike and I had obtained while studying normal and denervated cardiac ganglion cells. We had obtained evidence that the principal neurons in the ganglion were forming synapses with each other when they were deprived of their preganglionic inputs. This was of some interest since, at least in frogs, these neurons were not thought to interact synaptically in normally innervated ganglia. Most of our data were obtained by recording from individual neurons while stimulating large numbers of ganglion cells antidromically via the postganglionic nerve. We had tried unsuccessfully on a few occasions to record simultaneously from pairs of neurons and demonstrate synaptic interaction directly. The problem was that the presynaptic cell might be any of a thousand neurons in the preparation, only a few of which are in the same field as the target cell. We weren't worried about the origin of the "intrinsic" synaptic inputs in chronically denervated ganglia, though, since the principal cells were supposed to be the only

81

neurons in the ganglion. After presenting these arguments to Steve, he asked something on the order of "Why don't you do the direct experiment?" I explained that we had tried a few times, and I recounted all the reasons why we might not be successful with additional effort. Steve's nonverbal reaction to all this was that the work would be made or broken, in his mind, by whether the "direct experiment" was done. Unless we could demonstrate by recording from pairs of neurons that ganglion cells had formed synapses with each other, then, for Steve, the result would remain in the "interesting, if true" category (into which, rumor has it, Steve also placed the Bible). Ultimately, Mike and I were able to demonstrate directly, in three instances, that ganglion cells had made synapses with one another in chronically denervated ganglia. This required testing about 700 pairs of neurons (we stopped with the pair which yielded the third example), but it was certainly worth the effort.

Steve's ability to devise the "direct experiment" and to perform it with elegance is evident throughout his published work. He was consistently able to slice through to the core of the problem and to formulate the revealing experiment or experiments that ought to be done. We are all the better for this talent, both for what it has done to the field of neurobiology and for its having rubbed off on many of us.

Colin A. Nurse
Department of Biology
McMaster University
Hamilton, Ontario, Canada

In the summer of 1971 I first met Steve Kuffler during the early days of my graduate training in neurobiology. With my engineering background and relatively little exposure to biology, I had only recently read about Steve in Bernard Katz's text, *Nerve, Muscle and Synapse*, which, in addition to providing the usual grounding for aspiring neurobiologists, flashed occasional glimpses of the broad range of Steve's contribution to neurobiology and of his international prominence and stature. The details of our initial meetings are only sketchy, but what was memorable early on was that instead of meeting someone who by all accounts should be satisfied and content with an already fulfilling career, I found an amiable mentor and energetic scientist who still had the vigor to pursue research with both curiosity and enjoyment but without sacrificing a firm commitment to excellence. With remarkable insight he had already built a department of which he was chairman and which for many years after remained at the forefront of modern neurobiology. Though he may not have cared for the everyday duties of the chair, he managed to create around him a rich and exciting atmosphere in which graduate students, postdoctoral fellows, staff, and faculty intermingled freely.

As a graduate student I remember seeking Steve's advice on a few personal issues, and that he gave with genuine interest, concern, and sensitivity. As a colleague he was always easily approachable, yet he remained frank and constructive in criticism. I guess the event I cherished most and which for me provided true testimony to his character occurred a couple of years after my graduation. On a return trip to Harvard I was discussing my current research with Steve. He recognized that two of his colleagues, who I did not know personally at the time, would best be able to advise me on the particular problem. Steve went out of his way and invited me to dinner with him so I could discuss the problem with his colleagues. Some 11 years later I thank you for that memory, Steve.

Ann E. Stuart
Department of Physiology
University of North Carolina
Chapel Hill, North Carolina

From 1968 to 1971, and again from 1973 to 1979, owing to a generous quirk of fate rather than my own good judgment, I was part of Steve Kuffler's "family" at Harvard Medical School. I was at a life stage that was both too old and too young to fully appreciate Steve Kuffler's genius. I say too old, because his essence seemed instantly grasped by children, who were drawn to him as if by Pied Piper magic. If only every department chair would take off their shoes at departmental holiday parties and unabashedly run around with the children, daring them to pick up Coke bottles with their toes! I was too young to really know him at a peer level and, worse, too young to realize that I should study his style—his diplomacy, and his unerring sense of right and wrong, of the important and unimportant, of what the next fundamental scientific problem would be. Now I can only ask myself in every crisis, "What would Steve have said, or done?" No doubt whatever it was, it would have solved the problem at hand quickly and with a twist of highly original humor.

But I was just the right age—a young, committed student, then a postdoc, then a junior faculty member without outside distractions—to profit immensely from his neurobiology department. The place was permeated with his style and example. Friday sherry at four o'clock in his office (later, Friday beer-plus-dinner as the department grew) included everyone: secretaries, technical staff, pre-Nobel laureates, students. Everyone came . . . and the resulting friendships formed, ideas generated, and collaborations planned are uncountable. Steve was always around—lab door open, always at lunch and beer hour—and so being around and friendly was the thing to do: I and many others literally lived in the lab, not because of a race with the competition but for the sheer joy of the experiments and the friendships. When Steve found a noon seminar intriguing he might stay and question the speaker until 2:00 or 3:00 P.M., and what student could miss the message that outstanding science ran on honest curiosity, not a schedule? Steve's encouragement of me and all of us young scientists was continuous: often he would wander into my lab and ask to look at a preparation or watch an experiment for awhile. And so the normal structure of departments became reversed in this one, with the students getting first priority on the technical services, and the younger faculty the favored teaching. Not only that, it was his unstated assumption that whatever anyone in his department was working on was valuable, important, and worth everyone's time and attention. Thus the periodic "evening meetings," even for beginning students presenting their first few experiments, were a time of excitement and thrill. Steve's humor, ranging from puns to obscure jokes, percolated throughout the department—I have never been certain whether he simply selected people with a good sense of humor who then chose others of similar nature, or whether he inspired a humor competition within the group, but there it was—laughter at every turn. Laughter, and intensely serious intellectual effort—primarily but not entirely in neurobiology: inspired by Steve's wide-ranging curiosity, the department's lunchtime seminar menu occasionally offered up professionals in such different fields as calligraphy and black holes.

Now that I have a child, I see Steve more clearly, for what delights me in my child and his friends are the same qualities that delighted me about Steve: uncontaminated curiosity, friendliness without suspicion of hidden intent, playfulness, intense work on an idea for the pure joy of it, the absence of ulterior motive, and, somehow, the clear perception of right and wrong.

Paul H. Patterson
Division of Biology
California Institute of Technology
Pasadena, California

I very much appreciate the opportunity to contribute some thoughts on Steve. My most valued memories of Steve are related to his lively, informal style and his ready sense of humor. Although I arrived as a junior person, he readily accepted me (and, in turn, my students, postdocs, and technicians) as a valued member of the Harvard Neurobiology Department family. He set a tone of friendliness and camaraderie, and one could not help but respond in kind. The lack of pompous, authoritarian rule of the department was marvelous for the community. I have often wondered about the spirit of rigorous, yet congenial, scholarly adventure so palpably present in all of our social and intellectual gatherings of those days—how much of it was due to Steve's own style, and how much was due to the personalities of the remarkable group of faculty he put together?

What did he think of this extraordinary assemblage that he had created? A visitor to the department inquired along these lines, asking, "How many people are working in your department?" Characteristically, Steve answered, "About half."

Dale Purves
Department of Neurobiology
Duke University Medical Center
Durham, North Carolina

I met Steve Kuffler during my first year of medical school when, as a freshman with no particular interest in the nervous system, I took what was then called "Area III." This was a course of three or four weeks that introduced us to neurobiology. Steve's faculty included Ed Furshpan, Dave Potter, Ed Kravitz, Dave Hubel, and Torsten Wiesel. Naive though we were, we recognized the tremendous intellectual strength of this contingent; even those who thought the subject matter too esoteric for a career in plastic surgery or dermatology were deeply impressed by the fact that the faculty, at Steve's behest, knew each student's name.

Seven years later when, as a first year neurosurgery resident, I decided to try my own hand at research, I had the sense to seek Steve's advice. He suggested I would do well to work with John Nicholls, who was just then returning to Steve's department from Yale. In the two years I spent as a postdoc with John, and during the subsequent year with Jack McMahan, I got to see at first hand the aspects of Steve's personality that made him so influential. To a beginning postdoc woefully ignorant of neuroscience, Steve was eminently reassuring. Not only was he genuinely considerate, but more importantly, he had no desire to intimidate the uninitiated. His straightforward, even simplistic, approach encouraged us to think the body of information we were trying to absorb might actually be tractable. In short, we students were buoyed up in our labors by the remarkable success of an intellect that Steve made seem not all that different from our own.

Steve further endeared himself by an obvious enjoyment in deflating colleagues who had a more glorious view of themselves than he thought warranted. One day a prominent visitor from Europe was delivering a very long-winded lunchtime seminar. After an hour and a half, the lecturer was only halfway through a second carousel of slides, and the audience was visibly restive. Steve, who was sitting as usual in the back of the lunchroom where these seminars were held, leaned over to Mary Hogan, his longtime friend and technician, and told her to advance the carousel to the last few slides. With some trepidation (but doubtless relief) Mary obeyed. The lecturer, who gave no sign of having noticed the abridgement, concluded promptly as the final few slides appeared in order on the screen.

In spite of the general spirit of camaraderie, and the first-name basis which Steve insisted upon in his dealings with virtually everyone in the department, I don't think any of us at my level were really close to him. In a way, that was useful. A leader of Steve's caliber balances the student's need for fellowship with enough distance to allow a degree of reverence. This art Steve mastered exactly.

John Hildebrand
Arizona Research Laboratories
Division of Neurobiology
The University of Arizona
Tucson, Arizona

To be a postdoc in the Department of Neurobiology at Harvard Medical School in the late 1960s and early 1970s was a wonderfully stimulating and exhilarating experience, especially for those of us who came from other areas of science to "cut our teeth" in the emerging field of neurobiology. We found ourselves immersed in an extraordinary community of physiologists, anatomists, and biochemists—established investigators working next to green recruits—in which the unwritten code of conduct combined scientific rigor, honesty, and single-minded, uncompromisingly hard work with generous collegiality, cohesive group spirit, open communication, and full-blooded fun. Unobtrusively presiding over this unique "family" was Steve Kuffler, its founder, paterfamilias, and chief punster. He was always one of the first to welcome newly arrived students and postdocs, and he went out of his way to grant them kindness, interest, and concern. Not the least important example of that warmth were the Thanksgiving gatherings in their home to which Phyllis and Steve invited students and postdocs—especially those who were alone.

In retrospect, I realize that Steve led by setting an example and lending tone to the group. His playfulness, which had its highest expression in his deadly puns and fractured jokes, helped to foster cordial, comfortable feelings and relations among the members of the department. At the frequent lunchtime seminars, he never hesitated to ask "dumb" questions that broke the ice, emboldened others, and sometimes revealed much about the speaker or his work. Steve did not conceal his passion for his experiments, his reactions to ideas and manuscripts, or his disdain for pompousness, vanity, and stupidity. He was uncannily adept at juggling his scientific and administrative activities, getting his colleagues to shoulder responsibilities, and making people feel good about the department. Although he always gave top priority to his own scientific work and eschewed distractions, he clearly cared deeply about the welfare of the department and his faculty colleagues, and I believe that he quietly took considerable pride in their successes.

Near the end of my postdoctoral fellowship, I learned once and for all that Steve was the grand master of the zinger. The chairman of a developing department in a developing university had offered me a faculty position at a surprisingly advanced rank, with numerous tantalizing privileges. At once dazzled and puzzled by this overly generous offer, I went to Steve for advice. I outlined the situation for him and expressed my uncertainty about what to do. After a short pause, and eyeing me with a twinkle over the top of his glasses, Steve asked me: "Do you really want to take that job?" I mumbled something about my reluctance to do it despite its glitter. Without a moment's hesitation, Steve shot back: "Well, then, it's very clear what you should do. Just tell them you're not that good!" That settled the matter for me, but I still have the vaguely uncomfortable feeling—one familiar to Steve's friends and colleagues—that I am not sure what he really meant by that amusing response.

The outcome of my search for a job was both unforeseen and fortunate. I chose the one offer that provided a small, empty lab, installed me in a cramped office (the small space and one telephone which I had to share with Paul Patterson for years), included no setup funds, substituted a hunting license for salary support in place of an institutional paycheck, and permitted no hope of eventual tenure. Nevertheless, it was unquestionably my great good fortune to become an Assistant Professor in the Department of Neurobiology at Harvard in 1972. It is hard to imagine a better context in which to be a junior faculty member and build a research program than that place at that time. I experienced many pleasures over the next eight years, but none meant more to me than my growing friendship with Steve Kuffler.

Among Steve's endearing qualities was his unpredictability. For example, he often walked into my lab when I least expected a visitor.

One instance comes to mind and is probably typical of what many of us experienced with him. I was working alone late one night, trying to complete a large number of difficult dissections. I was feeling very tired, frustrated, and sorry for myself. As I peered with bleary eyes through my operating microscope, I sensed that someone had approached close to my side. I grunted a half-greeting without looking up and was startled to hear Steve's voice reply. He asked about the experiments I was doing, said kind and supportive things to me, and really buoyed my spirits. Then, on the point of departing, he paused, gave me one of his inimitable looks, and said: "Just remember, John, these are the good old days!"

If such visits were characteristic, so were his oddly timed telephone calls. Once in a while, Steve would unexpectedly call me at home and propose a spontaneous outing together. I remember one such call, which awakened me about seven o'clock on a Sunday morning. Steve asked me what I was doing. Too embarrassed to tell him that he had got me out of bed, I said something about preparing breakfast. His reply was one that I had learned to expect at such times: he suggested that, if I wasn't planning to do anything else, we might have brunch together in the restaurant on top of the Prudential Center in Boston. His spirit of camaraderie meant a lot to me, and outings like that one with Steve were real treats.

One of my last interactions with Steve took place under similarly characteristic circumstances at the Marine Biological Laboratory in Woods Hole on a balmy August evening in the summer of 1980. A Friday night lecture had just ended, and, leaving Lillie Auditorium, I bumped into Steve on the front steps. He proposed that we retreat to his home for a beer or two, and off we went. What ensued was the most important and memorable experience I ever had with him. At the end of an unusually candid, widely ranging, and extended conversation, Steve grew very earnest. He spoke about the department he had built and led, about colleagues, about our ways of doing science in universities, and about leadership. Then he told me not to be afraid to go off on my own and build and lead my own group. By the time his messages really began to be clear to me, it was October, I was packing up to leave Harvard, and Steve was gone. His advice has helped me very much over the last decade, as I have tried to do just what he urged upon me. I wish only that I could have thanked him for that inspiration and for his many other gifts to me.

Kenneth J. Muller
Department of Physiology and Biophysics
University of Miami School of Medicine
Miami, Florida

I have many fond memories of Steve Kuffler, beginning in 1971 when I joined his department to work as a postdoc with John Nicholls and later with Jack McMahan. Already I was aware of the key role he played in guiding American neuroscience and felt fortunate to be able to watch firsthand his brilliant, but unassuming, approach to science. High standards and clever insights were his hallmarks. He always seemed to be looking at things from new angles, and I suppose even his puns were an indication of this. His plays on words and the twinkle in his eyes were also a part of his interactions with students and colleagues, for whom he showed warm regard. Work in the department was clearly stimulated and, in some cases, inspired by Steve.

Steve Kuffler's scientific gifts are well documented, and I am not the one to talk about historical aspects of the Neurobiology Department. I should instead like to describe two small incidents that reflect two aspects of Steve's human side—his regard for students and his physical agility.

Although Steve did not have students (except postdoctoral fellows) working in his lab, he treated even undergraduates with respect and seemed always ready to extend himself for students. One undergraduate I had gotten to know at M.I.T. came to the department one afternoon to hear a seminar. Steve noticed him alone in the hall, asked his name, and helped him to the seminar room. A few weeks later when the student returned, Steve greeted him by name and welcomed him back to the department. What an impact this had on the student, who then earned his doctorate in neurobiology.

Anyone who saw Steve on skis in the Harvard Forest or on the tennis court in Woods Hole had a sense of his physical agility, but I did not fully appreciate it until I saw Steve one evening at a Neurobiology Department party. In one game the contestants were required to stand behind a line, squat to grasp the end of an unopened can of vegetables on the other side of the line, and slide the can forward as far as possible, using the can and the toes for support. Steve was the winner. He slid the can out from the line, supported himself horizontally over the floor without touching it, his hands stretched over his head as far

90

as he could reach, grasping the end of the can. As if this were not enough, he gracefully slid the can back to the line, in a kind of extreme push-up, and then stood. I have never seen his match. The whole stunt was performed with typical Steve Kuffler flair and modesty.

It was a joy to have such sensitivities and talents in one person. I deeply miss Steve as a scientist and human being.

Darwin K. Berg
Department of Biology
University of California, San Diego
La Jolla, California

Steve Kuffler is a hero to me. He chose important issues, and with imagination, insight, and hard work revolutionized how people thought about them. He had a unique ability to develop powerful experimental systems that in his hands opened up entire fields of new research. Characteristically, he then left the rich opportunities that emerged for others to pursue while he chose the more difficult path of moving on to yet another area, identifying new questions and developing experimental approaches for them.

Steve was Chairman of the Department of Neurobiology at Harvard Medical School when I entered the field, first as a postdoctoral fellow there, too many years ago. Despite what must have been a considerable administrative burden, he seemed to make it invisible as he devoted long hours day after day to experiments. Steve inspired by example. His passion for science was obvious, and the rigor that he demanded of his own work set standards for us all.

It wasn't until many years later that I also came to recognize Steve's talent for creating a unique research climate. This extended to his selection of people, his shielding of people from administrative demands so that they were free to work, and his encouraging the kind of interactions among people that were constructive rather than competitive. I remember, for example, that when some of us became overly impressed with our own critical abilities in questioning seminar speakers, Steve would gently deflate our pretensions by volunteering questions such as, "Was that done with or without pH?" or suggesting that a particular question "had already been taken." Another perhaps

91

apocryphal remark I recall often attributed to Steve is that, "If you publish more than two papers a year you can't be taken seriously." Some of us take refuge in this; others hope he was referring only to some arcane division of neurophysiology.

Steve will also be remembered by many of us in another way. He seemed to care deeply about the success of young scientists and worked to help them thrive and do well. Often he played an instrumental role in advancing the career of an individual, and did so with such adroitness and modesty that the individual remained unaware of Steve's role for years. Those of us in La Jolla who knew Steve also remember with fondness and nostalgia the dinner or breakfast meeting that he would always arrange to bring us together when his many obligations brought him to our area. We miss him.

Monroe W. Cohen
Department of Physiology
McGill University
Montreal, PQ, Canada

This is a letter written to Steve by Monroe in 1973.

Dear Steve:

There are many fond memories that I have of the three wonderful years working with you. I must admit however that in some respects the beginning, like most beginnings, was difficult. I was not especially attracted to *Necturus* when you first introduced me to him. Nor did I derive much pleasure from the many times that I tried to follow your example of dissecting out his optic nerve and setting it up for experimentation only to find that I had reduced its diameter to 50 microns or irretrievably lost it in the suction electrode. But you continued to tell me that I was doing well and I began to believe you. I still floundered for many months with the problem of glial contribution to surface recordings and it was only as a result of your continued help and reassurance that it finally worked out so nicely. And in the meantime I became rather fond of our mud-hound with the stiff upper lip.

Having Hersch-Gersch join us to study the ionic environment of glial cells and neurons was a real delight. His philosophical excursions and repeated declarations that everyone and everything in the lab, including the animals, "are much too good for me" caused many good laughs. Somehow we also managed to get work done and one day you suggested that we ought to begin to write it up. The next morning Hersch and I were both flabbergasted when you gave us a full rough draft which turned out to require little revision.

A special highlight, for both Myrna and myself, was the wonderful interlude when you took me along to La Jolla to learn tissue culture à la Harrison in the summer of '67. From the beginning you exerted "le droit de seigneur" and made most, if not all, of the cultures yourself because they were novel and fun. But I learned a great deal, and the promising recordings that we made during the last week gave me a strong motivation for carrying on this work subsequently.

It is now eight years since you offered to take me on as a post-doctoral fellow. At that time I was a student in your neurophysiology course at Woods Hole, and you asked me why I was interested in working with you. I replied that it would be an honor. I don't believe I was being glib, for I was familiar with many of your publications, but it may have sounded so and in retrospect I have wondered whether my reply might have generated some second thoughts in your own mind. Of course, now I can say with much firmer conviction that it is, and was, an honor to work with you. But much more than that, it was for me a most instructive and rewarding experience. Not only because of the tangible scientific accomplishments but also because of the insights I was able to gain from seeing your approach to scientific problems and to people. Your warm generosity, humor and endless dedication will always remain a source of inspiration.

It is a deep pleasure for me to participate in this tribute to you on your 60th birthday. Happy birthday and many happy returns.

Michael J. Dennis
**Denman Island
British Columbia, Canada**

When I first arrived at H.M.S. Neurobiology as a newly fledged post-doctoral fellow, I was put into a holding tank with Hersch Gerschenfeld, there to probe and ponder the wonders of rat glial cells (the most delightful of colleagues and the most boring of subjects). During that period I was anxious as to whether or not I would be asked to work directly with Steve. In that condition I had the following dream:

> I am in the hall just outside Steve's office and lab at H.M.S. The surroundings are familiar except that I notice a door where I had not seen one before (such that it would let into the little cloakroom/toilet area behind Steve's office). Just then the door opens—inside I see an operating chair with a group of orderlies lifting off a small person wrapped from head to foot in white gauze, except for a bloody opening in the chest. The small homunculus person is kicking and screaming in protest as it is lifted. An orderly comes out with a pan of tissue (digits, jawbone, teeth, flesh). Someone beside me says, "Oh. Didn't you know Dr. Kuffler has for years performed experimental surgery on retarded children, with considerable success."

Not long after dreaming this Steve did ask me to work directly with him, to subject me to the corrections of his metaphorical surgery. He gave me valuable work skills which serve me still.

One of the strongest of the gifts he gave me was the habit of proceeding with caution, of being careful to have enough information before drawing conclusions, to be certain of what you were saying before you said it. Steve would never accept the experimental results that John Harris and I came up with until he too had performed the experiments and obtained them for himself. However, he did not want to be alone in the experimentation, he wanted company—he wanted mine. This was great, except that his time and desire for experimentation seemed often to fall on Friday in the late afternoon and carried into the evening. At that time, in the young adulthood of my childhood, I had other things on my mind besides microelectrodes and ACh sensitivity, especially on Friday night. I chafed as I sat behind him in the dark little room—I struggled internally, like the bound homunculus, figuratively castrated. Even then though, and still now, I respected that caution and thoroughness with which he proceeded.

Another domain in which Steve taught me a lot by his example was that of written communication. He knew how to accurately convey scientific information. His method was quite simple really, though painstaking, and even painful at times to the impatient neophyte. He, we, would consider every word of every sentence, stopping with each to ask if it conveyed the thought intended. We would go over, and over . . . and over, back and forth through a manuscript until it said exactly what we wanted to say, nothing more and nothing less. This was a laborious procedure. I remember tedious hours in his office with Jack McMahan and me rolling our eyes at one another, doing it Steve's way. At times I wanted to run from the room screaming. But I thank him now for that gift of precision.

It is ironic that as parents and mentors our task is to wean or wrest childhood away from our charges—to force them to conform to the dictates of society; to sit still, be quiet, be patient, work hard, be careful, and stop playing. In a sense this is what my dream foretold; this is what Steve did to me. Yet at the same time one of his most endearing traits was his own childish playfulness. He could be silly in a completely unself-conscious way, and then laugh at himself. Children loved him for it, as did the child in me. Our world needs more childish play, more freedom from vain pretense, such as that which Steve gave to us all.

Another, more problematic, area in which Steve tried to, and to some extent did, influence me was that of political activity. The period during which I worked with him, 1967–70, was the time of the war in Vietnam, of massive protest from the youth, and I was of that youth. Steve did not approve of such activity. I remember evenings of argument with Steve and Torsten about whether one should act to promote political change. Steve was firmly of the conviction that scientists should confine their attention to the pursuit of science, that it was a serious mistake to try to act politically as well. He recounted that in prewar Vienna he was horrified to find himself marching with a gun in a youth corps; then and there he vowed to himself he would never get involved with any political movement again. He and I never came to agreement on this issue, and I still disagree. Now more than ever it is essential for each of us, scientist and artist, to ask ourselves what we feel about the comportment of our government, of our society, and to act on our consciences. We as biologists must be concerned for the future of life on this planet.

Naturally, in my relationship with Steve I was concerned about his opinion of me, was anxious for his approval; I hoped that the father would like me, the mentor would respect me, the doctor would proclaim that my surgery had been successful. As is common in such relationships I never really felt that I got all of the approval/appreciation that I wanted. I was never really sure what he thought of me. I knew he liked me OK, but I wanted something more. When I last saw Steve, in San Francisco in 1980, I had decided to quit science and move to an island in British Columbia. I wanted to speak honestly and openly with him about my intentions, but I could not; I still feared his parental disapproval, his pronouncement that all that effort to correct my mental retardation had failed. So I talked about going away for a while, but I skirted complete openness. Then he flew off to La Jolla. A few days later I received a brief letter (copy enclosed) from him in which he sent the love and appreciation I had always wanted. He had sensed my intentions and sent me on my way with his approval.

I thank Stephen Kuffler again for all he gave us.

La Valencia Hotel
La Jolla, California
January 17. 80*
between SF and Boston flying high (as ~~always~~, sometimes)

Hi Mike, it was brief but good to see you yesterday. So nice that you have retained the essential characteristics that I always liked—no pretence, just being yourself. You have taught me a good deal and continue to do so—thanks. It's refreshing.

Hope that life on your island comes up to expectations, yours and Vickie's. You didn't talk about Laramie, so I guess she will divide her time as before.

> Best wishes, as always,
> (signed Steve)

*The entire note was handwritten.

Mike is now a sculptor. One of his sculptures was recently purchased by UCSF for display in a courtyard.

H. Criss Hartzell
The Heart Cell Laboratory
Department of Anatomy and Cell Biology
Emory University School of Medicine
Atlanta, Georgia

The most prominent memory that I have of Steve was during the summer of 1975 when we were at Woods Hole. Steve, Doju Yoshikami, and I were scheduled to give one of the Friday night seminars, and we were practicing our talks. Since these Friday night seminars were referred to as the "Friday night fights," I was reasonably nervous, anyway. As I began my practice talk, Steve interrupted my first sentence saying, "Are you going to start *that* way?" He wanted me to give some background before jumping into the data, whereas as a young postdoc I thought that everyone at Woods Hole certainly knew the background better than I did! Throughout my sojourn with Steve, he stressed the importance of placing an experiment in a physiological context and *explaining* its rationale. During that afternoon at Woods Hole, Steve and Doju continued to interrupt and make suggestions at a rate of what seemed to be twice per sentence. When I finished, completely exhausted, Steve suggested we convene in two hours so that I could practice the revised version! I really didn't know whether I could do it, but in retrospect it was probably the best learning experience of my life. It was certainly the most unforgettable!

Likewise, we would sit together for days at the large conference table in Steve's office, discussing the manuscripts we wrote word by word. It was agonizing, but Steve provided a rare example of someone who cared more about doing it properly than anything else. His caring for people was also the basis of his ruthlessness in making sure we did it right. I don't think Steve ever resorted to taking a shortcut, even if it meant that a paper didn't get finished. Steve could have written those manuscripts himself in a fraction of the time he spent agonizing with us. Steve could have given a better talk at Woods Hole than I did, even after two days of his coaching me, but he cared deeply about training the best scientists and doing the best research. I can think of no one I have ever known with as much integrity as Steve.

Stephen Roper
Department of Anatomy and Neurobiology
Colorado State University
Fort Collins, Colorado

Steve always cracked pistachio nuts beside me when we were trying to impale cardiac ganglion cells with micropipettes. It seemed he would wait until I was just about to insert an electrode poised just above the elusive neuron. Crack! Damn! Another poor impalement. We had been working several months attempting to confirm and extend the work Steve had just finished with Mike Dennis and John Harris on parasympathetic cardiac ganglion cells in the frog. But now we were exploring a more difficult preparation, multiply innervated ganglion cells in the *Necturus* heart. It seemed impossible to obtain stable impalements in this new preparation. Everything we tried to make decent microelectrodes for the *Necturus* cardiac neurons failed and Steve and I were on the verge of giving up on the mud-puppy preparation. Perseverance and stubbornness prevailed, though. The experiments eventually were successful and resulted in the study of ACh chemosensitivity and transmitter supersensitivity on partially denervated neurons. From this experience I learned a great deal from Steve about how to push hard on a methodology until the technological barriers give way and the underlying biological questions lie exposed.

I recall that Steve was forever searching for new preparations to explore. The objective was to find a bit of the nervous system that had a relatively simple cytological organization and that was exposed so that individual cells and their synaptic contacts could be seen in the living isolated tissue. Many was the trip I took to the local pet store in La Jolla during the summer of 1971 to bring back to the laboratory an odd assortment of exotic salamanders, lizards, toads, and alligators for dissection in search of a new tissue preparation. At the store the clerk would usually place my newly purchased "pet" into a small paper sack for transport "home." I would set this sack next to me for the short drive back to the Salk Institute. Once during one of these sojourns, I picked up a hitchhiker who was thumbing his way north up the highway. The fellow must have thought the brown paper bag between us contained my lunch, since the trip was during the noon break. The hitchhiker nearly leapt out the window when my "lunch" began to squirm and gnaw through the sack! It was important for Steve to be able to observe the dissected tissue under the microscope and see the neurons directly. This allowed him to orient recording and stimulating electrodes visually. I believe this experimental approach was a significant aspect of many of his successes. It allowed Steve and his colleagues to conduct detailed experiments on synapses and to obtain conclusive answers to important, fundamental questions. I have attempted to emulate this approach in my own studies on the nervous system.

But most significant was the sense of playfulness and boyish curiosity that Steve brought to the laboratory. I probably didn't appreciate this as much while I was a young postdoc in Steve's laboratory, but I can now understand the importance of it. No question, however naive or simple, was ruled out with Steve. His straightforward questions sometimes caught us "hotshot" postdocs and students unprepared and exposed the thin ice upon which we had built some elaborate hypothesis. Experiments were intriguing games to Steve. Solving a puzzle about a bit of the nervous system was never tedious for Steve Kuffler. Several years back when he was a distinguished visitor at the University of Colorado Medical School, Professor Bernard Katz added a coda to his lecture with an introspective remark that neuroscience research above all must be fun . Steve's career and his successes epitomized this. Perhaps Steve was just funning me with the pistachios.

Doju Yoshikami
Department of Biology
University of Utah
Salt Lake City, Utah

I had a dream recently that featured Steve and about half a dozen or so faculty, postdocs, and students from his department during the '70s. They were clustered around his electrophysiological setup and all working excitedly on one experiment! In real life at any given time during an experiment Steve would have at most only two other "copilots"—any more than that wouldn't fit around his setup. Furthermore, in real life many of the investigators in the dream did not actually collaborate directly with each other on experiments. So this was one of those surreal scenarios typical of dreams. The details have

99

faded, but in the lingering images I see a reflection of one of Steve's many impressive accomplishments; that is, how he cultivated a superb environment, in his lab as well as his department as a whole, where individuals with diverse personalities and interests not only helped, but inspired one another.

When I started as a postdoc in Steve's lab in the early '70s I had no previous experience in neurobiology. However, Steve had attracted individuals like himself who were very approachable and willing to share their knowledge and expertise, and I had the good fortune of having as tutors not only Steve, but his colleagues as well. (One might wonder why Steve took me on when I had no training in neurobiology. Well, it was because he appreciated keenly that progress in neurobiology would be accelerated by infusing the field with researchers with diverse scientific backgrounds and perspectives.) My first tutor in neurobiology was Jack McMahan, who patiently instructed me how to perform dissections and how to use the microscope, and taught me histological techniques. Later Steve Roper introduced to me the basics of electrophysiology, from pulling electrodes to operating electronic instruments. A few experiments with Eric Frank on the physiology of the neuromuscular junction drew me more and more into electrophysiology, and one day I found myself at a setup with Steve himself.

One of the more fun experiments I did with Steve was the "ball-drop" series where we suspended in oil minute (~1/2 nl) droplets of Ringer's solution containing various concentrations of acetylcholine, and applied them to individual endplates of muscle fibers whose membrane potentials were monitored with intracellular microelectrodes. These experiments required five micromanipulators to position various microelectrodes and micropipettes while they were viewed with a compound microscope. Performing the experiments felt like piloting some craft. This experience gave me a special appreciation of how adept Steve was at flying by the seat of his pants, both physically and mentally. To be sure there were moments in these as well as other experiments when things didn't go well or got tedious. But Steve was always in good spirits, always level-headed. It was great working with Steve, no question about it. He had all one could ask for in a friend and collaborator: humor, humility, compassion, dedication, and an uncanny intuition. We joked a lot and constantly made puns. When Steve fumbled a punch line, that somehow made a joke all the more hilarious. Oh, those were the days!

To be sure I'll have more dreams about Steve—dreams reliving (and no doubt embellishing) seven wonderful years during which I had the privilege of working with him and his colleagues. I love him, and I miss him.

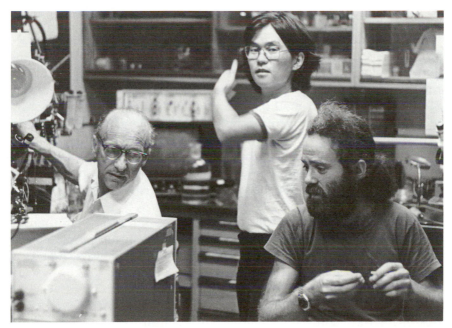

"The Maestro" with Doju Yoshikami (center) and Robert Stickgold in 1977. Photograph by Bob Bosler.

John P. Horn
Department of Physiology
University of Pittsburgh School of Medicine
Pittsburgh, Pennsylvania

I was a postdoctoral fellow in Steve Kuffler's lab during the last two years of his life. In early 1979, I arrived in Boston, filled with the enthusiasm and confidence of one who has just completed a Ph.D. In retrospect, my view of neurobiology was narrow. The environment in Steve's lab expanded my horizons and challenged me to grow as a scientist. He interested me in an important problem, guided me in my experimental approach, and then gave me the freedom to make my own discoveries. Although some days were difficult, it was a wonderful time. In this regard, I believe my experience was typical of many before me. It was good fortune to share in Steve Kuffler's legacy as a teacher of experimental biology.

During the last phase of his career, Steve's interests were focused upon the physiology of slow synaptic transmission in autonomic ganglia and the identification of peptide cotransmitters. As always, he was at the forefront of neurobiology. Initially, I was attracted to Steve's work by the papers that he and his colleagues had published on the synaptic physiology of the parasympathetic cardiac ganglion. After arriving in Boston, it took some time before I fully appreciated the beautiful balance in Steve's work on slow potentials between new ideas and older themes that could be traced back to much earlier experiments. Amongst the recurrent themes were the localization of synaptic receptors, the mimicry of synaptic potentials by exogenous agents, the functional role of acetylcholinesterase, and the discovery of new transmitters and their modes of action. Steve was influential both as a master of experimental technique and of scientific writing. The figures in his papers do not merely present data, they tell complex tales in simple and elegant terms. Preparing figures and text to meet his standards was an exasperating task that remains the substance of folklore.

As a mentor, Steve was straightforward and deceptively simple. Although demanding, he was fair. He never gave explicit instructions for projects. Instead, experimental ideas were presented as seemingly innocent suggestions. In this way, I began to investigate the muscarinic inhibition of sympathetic neurons. My respect and admiration for Steve grew from the realization that he expected no more from others than of himself. Watching him in the lab, it was obvious that he loved to dissect preparations and poke cells. Although his eyesight was poor by that time, he would not be deflected from the obvious enjoyment that he obtained by making preparations. When impaling a cell, he tapped at selected spots on the manipulators and table with the care and touch that one associates with a virtuoso sitting at an old familiar piano. To indulge his passion for experimenting, he worked long hours and guarded his time. In a letter that I received shortly before arriving in Boston, he said "We expect to have fun in the lab and, I hope, outside of the lab. We can arrange other matters after I get back from Woods Hole." That summer, Lily and Yuh-Nung Jan and Steve discovered the transmitter role of LHRH in frog sympathetic ganglia. At one point during my first few months in the lab, I began to stray from the goals of my project because it was difficult and I was frustrated with the lack of progress. Rather than point out the faults in my diversionary experiments, Steve simply reminded me of the original questions that we had discussed. He was fond of saying that you could pull a noodle, but you couldn't push it. Upon returning to my original project, things began to work. Steve immediately showed interest and encouraged me further. Months later, on a Friday afternoon, the day before Steve died, we had a lively conversation in the lab, then he drove down to Woods Hole for the weekend. Steve talked with greater than usual excitement about plans for future experiments, things that he thought we should test, and new postdocs joining the lab in the future. On that Sunday I learned the shocking news of his sudden death. After speaking about it with Jane Dodd, my collaborator and close colleague in the lab, we spent the afternoon wandering aimlessly around Boston trying to recover our senses. Comfort came from the knowledge that Steve had gone swimming in the Atlantic on that final October afternoon and that he was vitally engaged in his love of synaptic physiology until the end.

AFTER THE END

I returned to my home at Stanford around midnight to find a note saying Steve had died from a heart attack after swimming at Woods Hole. I immediately left on the "red-eye" flight to Boston and, assuming that the action would be at Woods Hole, took the earliest bus to the Cape, arriving there in late morning. It was one of those October days that couldn't make up its mind whether it was going to be cloudy or sunny, chilly or balmy. I shuffled through the leaves the mile from the bus depot to Steve's house. Oddly, my first reaction had been, "How could he do this to us?" Now I felt sad and empty.

The atmosphere at the house was frenetic. Numerous friends had dropped in to offer condolences. Several of the boys were there, frantically looking up numbers and calling on the telephone to notify colleagues throughout the world what had happened. They also were to contact The New York Times *and* The Boston Globe *to place an obituary, to wait anxiously while* The Times *contacted its people in New York City to determine whether Steve was noteworthy, and, after the O.K. was given, to work desperately to write the obituary before the deadline. Almost ludicrously, there were brief arguments over such trivial things as whose work with Steve would be and would not be mentioned. And while this was going on, Phyllis and those of the children who were already there sat or moved in stunned silence. A glimpse told me that I would be of no value here, and so I spent the rest of the day shuffling through the leaves, visiting places where Steve and I had walked and talked.*

Hearing him say:

"ooooooooohhhh . . . . " in excitement over a beautiful preparation.

"We're tired . . . but a good kind of tired," after a long night's work.

"You must learn when not to listen to me," after bringing me to his point of view.

"It's those damned harps again, isn't it?" indicating that one could find something to complain about even in heaven.

Already missing his lengthy phone calls at midnight or early in the morning that began with, "Whatcha doin' Jack?" and wound up with me feeling much better about almost everything than I had before he called.

Thinking about his advice when I left for Stanford a few years before:

"Don't try to do everything."

"You can't make everybody happy."

"If you don't want to do something, do it poorly and people won't ask you again."

"You have to select students carefully. A bad student is worse than none at all. The bad ones will slow you down and eventually from their own frustration will tear you apart."

"It doesn't matter how smart someone is; if he's not fun to have around, it isn't worth it."

"Take care of your research and it will take care of you."

Worrying about his doubts:

"Even at this age I still think about quitting. What we do is really hard."

"I probably should have stuck to just one thing. Probably the visual system . . . but the guys were already into the visual cortex and well . . . you know . . . ."

That evening, Torsten and I drove back to Boston together, tired and depressed. During the first part of the ride we were almost totally silent. In the middle part we began reminding each other of Stevenisms and found ourselves at times chuckling almost uncontrollably. Finally, in a silly sort of way, we began to wonder what would happen to neuroscience now that Steve was no longer at the helm. Would the charlatans and self-promoting lightweights take over? Would serious science be replaced by a blizzard of hype and exciting but untestable hypotheses?

Of course things are probably no different now than they were then, there is just more (except grant money). But if we could ask Steve what he thought about the current state of neuroscience he would probably respond with one of his puzzling phrases like, "Things didn't turn out half bad," accompanied by a twinkle in his eye.

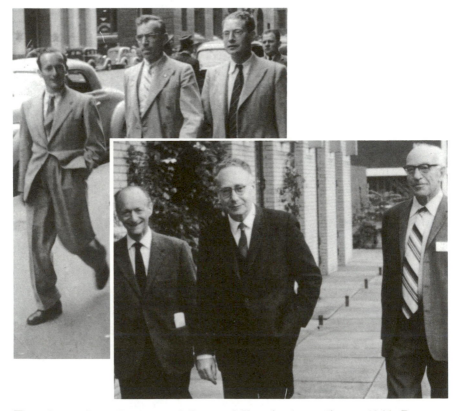

Top: Steve, John Eccles, and Bernard Katz in Australia ca. 1941. Bottom: Steve, Katz, and Eccles ca. 1975.

STEPHEN WILLIAM KUFFLER

24 August 1913 — 11 October 1980

Elected For.Mem.R.S. 1971

By SIR BERNARD KATZ, F.R.D.

STEPHEN KUFFLER who died at his home in Woods Hole, Massachusetts, at the age of 67, was much beloved and admired, as a scientist and as a personal friend, by colleagues and pupils all over the world. He was acknowledged as one of the leading neurophysiologists of his generation whose work illuminated many different aspects of our nervous system and who by his brilliant experimental skill often achieved results that gave aesthetic as well as intellectual satisfaction. He died suddenly, at the height of his scientific activities. Though his close friends had warnings for many years of his precarious state of health, he had borne serious illness, glaucoma, cataract, several eye operations, diabetes, heart trouble, without complaint, with no sign of losing his cheerful disposition or his seemingly flippant sense of humour, and certainly without letting it interfere with his great pleasure in making experiments or even with his athletic hobbies, swimming and tennis.

ORIGIN AND CHILDHOOD

He left few notes about his early life (see Appendix II) and much of the following is compiled from information I received from his family and friends.

He was born on a country estate in Hungary where he spent the first 10 years of his life. His birth certificate describes him as Wilhelm (or Vilmos in Hungarian) Kuffler, born 24 August 1913 at the village of Táp, son of Wilhelm Kuffler, landholder, 27 years and Elsa Kertész, 25 years. Parents and son belonged to the reformed (Calvinist) church; this was quite common among the Hungarian landed gentry, who after the Reformation had turned Protestant to demonstrate a degree of independence from the Catholic Habsburg dynasty.

These entries in his birth certificate differ in a curious way from what we knew of him, and there are certain ambiguities about his choice of first name, his nationality and even his religious denomination. He evidently did not care much for 'Wilhelm' or William and preferred the name Stephen which he adopted in 1938 at the time of his emigration from Austria. It is not quite clear whether to consider Stephen as Hungarian or Austrian by origin, and he would probably have regarded the question as irrelevant in any case. It appears that, when the Habsburg empire was dismantled in 1919, Stephen's family opted for Austrian nationality. Later on, after his emigration, he became a 'stateless' person until he acquired British (Australian), and, finally, United States citizenship. As to his religious affiliation, he was brought up in the Roman Catholic faith, and was probably not aware himself of his Calvinist origin until he happened to examine his birth certificate in adult life. I do not know whether Stephen was ever a deeply religious person; my own impression was that his attitude towards the demands of his church was one of peaceful acquiescence rather than strong conviction, and even this may

108

have diminished as he became more fully absorbed by science. But there is no doubt that his Catholic connections had a most important influence on his life and the direction of his academic career, especially through the social contacts and personal associations they brought him after he left his native country, in particular meeting Jack Eccles in Sydney who gave him a start in physiology in 1938, and Phyllis Shewcroft whom he married in 1943.

In a brief biographical essay, Stephen speaks about his early life. 'I spent the first ten years of my life in Hungary on a medium-sized farm. My most vivid memories are about riding horses, swimming in ponds and occasionally visiting a nearby "big" city. At home we spoke Hungarian and German and learned reasonably good French from a succession of governesses.' The description of his home is probably an understatement. According to other accounts, it was quite a large estate with most of the villagers being employed on it; it housed a beautiful mansion surrounded by a magnificent park, replete with stables, ponies and grooms for Stephen and his two sisters, Elizabeth and Margaret. It was an idyllic existence which continued even after the tragic death of his mother from typhoid fever in 1918. The father (who was the eldest of six brothers) was running the estate as well as owning valuable property in Austria and in the capital, Vienna; he was an agricultural expert who had studied and obtained his academic diploma at the School of Agriculture in Berlin. After the mother's death, an Austrian lady together with a younger German assistant were engaged to look after the family; this arrangement worked very satisfactorily for the next few years until the father remarried and his new wife, Margit, a young widow with two daughters, took over the running of the home. The family life continued to be very happy, with 'nice memories of huge Christmas trees, mountains of toys and outings on horseback' (Margaret Wilmot's account). The final addition to the family was another girl, Marian, a half-sister to Stephen.

SCHOOL

The idyllic country life came to a final and sudden end in 1923 when Stephen was sent to a boarding school at Kalksburg outside Vienna, a classical type of 'gymnasium' run by Jesuits, which enjoyed a high reputation both for its scholastic attainments and for the humane and fairly liberal spirit which prevailed in spite of the strictly conservative religious tradition. This was, however, not the first traumatic interruption in Stephen's early life style. In the summer of 1919, during the short-lived communist regime of Béla Kun, the family had to make a quick escape across the Austro-Hungarian border, and I am told that the 6-year-old boy experienced a gun being pressed in his neck by some commissar who interrogated him about his father, who was already in Austria. It must have taught him a lesson which he put to use 19 years later, when he decided not to delay his departure (that time from Austria to Hungary)!

At Kalksburg, Stephen found himself in an entirely new environment and at first without the necessary preparation. 'A few attempts in elementary education on a private basis by the local school teacher [at Táp] had ended in complete failure.' The teachers at the boarding school decided very wisely to give Stephen a year of preliminary education to let him make up for his missing elementary schooling. After that, he took the full 8-year course which consisted of much Latin and Greek 'and practically no Science'. From accounts of one of his schoolmates, he was good, but not outstanding, did well in academic subjects and also at his favourite sports, swimming and tennis. He was popular and well-liked by his contemporaries, but apparently showed a certain restraint in his human relations which prevented the formation of close friendships.

UNIVERSITY

When Stephen left Kalksburg in 1932, his training at the gymnasium with its emphasis on linguistic studies had given him a bias towards the humanities or law. Nevertheless, for practical reasons and because of its international application he decided to go in for medicine at the University of Vienna. His progress is probably best described in his own words (see Appendix II), to which I add a few annotations. The University entrance requirements at that time, in Germany and Austria, were very simple: anyone with an 'Abitur' (high school leaving examination) had the right to enter the Faculty of his choice at any University, and one could also switch courses from one academic institution to another. Students who took up medicine or science, but came from a traditional type of classical 'gymnasium', received their basic scientific training in the first 2 years at the University. It was a matter of luck whether this training was inspiring and given by a teacher of great scientific achievements or by someone who regarded his lectures as an undesirable chore; in any case the student had much freedom of choice and could decide for himself which courses he wished to attend. There could be great advantages in being taught elementary science, for the first time, by an outstanding University teacher (I recall, as a junior medical student coming from a 'humanistic' school, receiving a memorable course of lectures and demonstrations in basic physics, given by P. Debye every day from 8 to 9 a.m.); but Stephen evidently did not have this kind of experience and, from his account, he seems to have suffered from a lasting feeling of inferiority in scientific and theoretical matters. But I was surprised to read of the 'almost unbearable challenge' of working with his seemingly more sophisticated colleagues (Appendix II); our working relations, at the time he refers to, were close and of the most friendly kind, with our daily experiments being accompanied by hilarious banter and almost competitive high-speed production of jokes and atrocious puns!

The year after Stephen started on his medical course, his father suffered a catastrophic financial reverse, and from then was unable to support him. Soon afterwards, the father died as a result of a stroke. Stephen received some help from his uncle Paul Kuffler, which enabled him to save enough for his travels abroad, but he had to finance himself by tutoring high-school boys and generally live with utmost economy.

For a time he left the students' hostel in Vienna and gave up his membership of a catholic students' society to take up residence in the house of his employer outside Vienna, as a family tutor. Even so, he managed to spend a summer vacation in the German Hospital in London and to hitch-hike to Egypt where his sister Elizabeth was working as a dentist in Cairo and where he also made the first acquaintance of the author John Brophy with whose family he formed very close ties.

In his final year at the University he rushed through his twelve clinical examinations, finishing them in record time and obtaining his M.D. in December 1937. Thereafter he worked for 3 months as an unpaid assistant at the 2nd Medical University Clinic and at the same time in the Institute of Pathology. As an undergraduate, pathology had been his favourite subject; for physiology he had no liking at all!

In his personal notes Stephen tells us some of the reasons which made him leave Austria after the 'Anschluss'. I understand there were additional, and probably more compelling factors, and I have taken the opportunity of discussing them with his closest colleague among his fellow students. He had been involved, though not very actively, with a conservative anti-Nazi group of students who had been planning some form of resistance against the Hitler invasion. They even possessed a small quantity of arms, but as with many of the other 'paramilitary' formations, it came to nothing, the police confiscated the weapons one day after the German troops had invaded Austria, and fortunately a sympathetic police officer destroyed the membership list which had come into his possession. Stephen was not aware of this last, very important circumstance, and, having been asked to report to the police the next day, he decided to make his getaway immediately. He had no difficulties in crossing the Hungarian border, as he had the necessary papers enabling him to make periodic visits to his old home. From Hungary he proceeded to England via Trieste, and after 3 months earning some money as a kind of companion (cum-teacher-cum-chauffeur) at a country mansion near Manchester and spending some time with his great friends the Brophys in London, he went by boat to Australia.

It appears that he greatly resented having to leave Vienna, and although many of his friends and acquaintances suffered political persecution under the Nazis, political reasons were probably not the primary motive for his emigration. His paternal grandmother came from a Jewish family, and he of course realized that this was quite enough to make life most unpleasant, if not impossible, under the new rulers of Austria. His uncle Paul who had helped him during the difficult undergraduate period was forced into labour service by the Nazis and died during the war.

AUSTRALIA

Stephen Kuffler arrived in Sydney in the summer of 1938. He met Professor Keith Inglis who had recently been appointed Head of the Pathology Department at Sydney University. (Before then, Inglis had been the first Director of the new Kanematsu Memorial Institute of Pathology at Sydney Hospital, and in 1937 was succeeded in this post by Dr J. C. Eccles, the well-known neurophysiologist—former Rhodes scholar from Melbourne who had worked with Sherrington at Oxford for many years before returning to Australia.) Inglis offered Kuffler an appointment as a demonstrator in Pathology, but it was an unpaid job, and his savings must have been dwindling at an alarming rate. He kept it up for 2 weeks and had the great fortune of being introduced, by a Jesuit priest Fr Richard Murphy, to Jack Eccles who, at the time, was looking for somebody who could give him a regular good game of tennis, and perhaps also make himself useful in the laboratory. Stephen seemed to have the right qualifications, at least for the former role.

Although Eccles had been appointed officially as Head of a Pathology Institute at a large general hospital, it was understood that he would not be required to direct the routine pathological work, and he was given a separate floor at the top of the building where he could establish a research laboratory in the field of his personal choice. He had support grants from the Australian Medical Research Council and was able to offer Stephen a junior post and encouraged him to join in his electro-physiological experiments which at that time were concerned with neuromuscular transmission.

During the first 12 months, Stephen found the subject bewildering and not without reason, for the interpretations placed on some of the electrical records were as confusing as the accompanying terminology; entities had been postulated (the so-called 'detonator response') for which no visible evidence could be produced, and it took a few years to eradicate them from the literature. When I arrived on the scene, in 1939, I could sense that Stephen had not yet come to terms with physiology, and for another year or so, I was wondering whether he would make it his career. If I had any beneficial influence, it was probably my reluctance to join Eccles and Kuffler in their mammalian experiments. Their work was done entirely on *in situ* recording from the anaesthetized whole cat; Stephen was very good in setting up this type of preparation, while I was not and did not even like it. Bringing with me the tradition of A. V. Hill's laboratory where most experiments were done on isolated tissue preparations of cold-blooded animals, I managed to persuade Stephen that there were certain advantages in working on simple systems, especially for the study of cellular and single synaptic processes. For a change, we introduced some nice Australian tree frogs (*Hyla aurea*) into the laboratory whose isolated nerve-sartorius preparations were just as suitable for long-lasting experiments as those of the English *Rana temporaria* to which I had been accustomed. I still remember Stephen roaring with laughter when I showed him how to 'take the frog's trousers off', a procedure which I mistakenly thought was known to every medical student. The laughs were on my side when I saw Stephen take his first sartorius muscle and place it into a beaker of hyposulphite instead of Ringer's solution. The real turning point in Stephen's career came a year later, in March or April 1941, when with Eccles's encouragement he pursued the isolation technique much further and produced the first work on a single isolated synapse; this will be described in the experimental section below. This was his first solo performance as a physiologist, and it immediately established his international reputation as a first-class experimenter. An article by Renshaw in the *Annual Review of Physiology* of 1943 already singles out Kuffler's 'beautiful experiments' on the isolated neuromuscular junction, and his series of papers in the *Journal of Neurophysiology* starting in 1942 were impressive enough for him to be appointed a National Research Council Fellow in Sydney (1943–45) and for R. W. Gerard to invite him in 1944 to take up a Seymour Coman Fellowship in Physiology at the University of Chicago.

Another event that was of importance for his subsequent career was the arrival in Sydney of Major A. M. Harvey, who had come with a group of medical officers from Baltimore to establish a field hospital for American soldiers in a Sydney suburb. Harvey's research interests, before he became Professor of Medicine at Johns Hopkins Medical School, had been in the field of neuromuscular transmission on which he had been working in Sir Henry Dale's laboratory in the 1930s. He re-established contact with Jack Eccles in Sydney, and this led to a fruitful collaboration with Stephen and to some joint papers on applied electrophysiology in humans. Stephen became an honorary part-time consultant with the U.S. Medical Corps during that period and, what was more important, A. M. Harvey got to know him well enough to arrange for Stephen to be offered a position at Johns Hopkins University in 1947.

Marriage and family

In April 1943 Stephen was married to Phyllis Shewcroft, who had just graduated from Sydney University Medical School. They had met first in April 1940, during some lectures which Eccles and I gave to the junior medical students in their Physiology course. Phyllis Kuffler, in addition to raising a family of four children, has had what one might call a multi-

113

disciplinary career: starting as an art student, then becoming a medical doctor and after their move to the United States acquiring expertise in educational psychology, with her particular interests in young persons' appreciation of visual arts and music. In these subjects she showed great enterprise, working with a youth orchestra and taking it on overseas tours, starting an art studio for young people, and teaching at the Rhode Island School of Design at Providence.

Their first child, Suzanne Elizabeth born in Sydney in 1945, is an artist currently working at Harvard Medical School. The other three were born in America, in 1947–49: Damien Paul, now a postdoctoral fellow in neurobiology at Stanford University; Julian Phillip, first teaching, then taking up medicine and now finishing his Internship at Maine Medical Center, and Eugenie Gabrielle who studied music in Paris and is active as a composer and performer.

MOVING TO THE UNITED STATES

In 1944, J. C. Eccles decided to leave, after some disagreement over policy questions with the administrators of Sydney Hospital, and to accept the Chair of Physiology at Otago University in New Zealand. Kuffler was able to continue his researches until 1945, but no prospects of a satisfactory appointment were in sight, and after obtaining his naturalization papers he applied for a United States visa to take up R. W. Gerard's invitation from Chicago University. This took some considerable time, and eventually an addendum had to be obtained to cover the newly arrived Suzanne as well as her parents. In the autumn of 1945, the Kuffler family finally departed by boat across the Pacific Ocean and settled for 15 months in Chicago. The initial period cannot have been easy, but it took Stephen very little time before he got down to some interesting work on the slow 'non-spiking' muscle fibres in the frog, and he quickly made friends with many American physiologists and with foreign postdoctoral visitors, in particular Yves Laporte from Toulouse (now at the Collège de France) who joined him under a French Government Research Fellowship in 1946. Stephen's move to Baltimore, to the Wilmer Institute of Ophthalmology at Johns Hopkins Medical School, is well described in his personal notes, where he refers to it as a 'wonderful place', with himself given charge of 'a small basement laboratory that soon became filled with a group of eager young postdoctoral workers, several of them from abroad, particularly Great Britain'. He stayed at Hopkins for 12 years, first as Associate Professor, later as Professor of 'Ophthalmic Physiology and Biophysics'. The first few years were a period of very close collaboration with C. C. Hunt, especially on muscle spindles and intrafusal motor innervation. Later came other important work, on the mammalian retina, more on nerve-muscle transmission in 'slow' fibres and on the stretch receptor neurons in Crustacea—some of it done at Woods Hole.

Kuffler's association with the Marine Biological Laboratory started in 1947; for many years the whole family used to spend the summer months at Woods Hole, at first being housed in a cottage close to the class rooms where he taught physiology and initiated a neurobiology training programme. Later they bought a house a few minutes away, near to the beach on Buzzard's Bay. Over the years, Stephen and Phyllis greatly improved and enlarged it. Stephen loved this house; it became to him a kind of dream home, a place of peace and refuge to which he returned even during the winter months when the laboratory and the village were almost deserted. There was an intermediate period starting in 1967, when Stephen and Phyllis decided to spend the summer vacations at La Jolla in Southern California and he was doing his summer work at the Salk Institute, but after 1971 he returned to his favourite summer residence at Woods Hole.

In a letter written in February 1958 to a distant cousin in South Africa, Stephen summarizes his Baltimore cum Woods Hole years as a very happy period for the whole family 'even after eleven years of it'. Johns Hopkins University had given him 'a generous appointment as Professor with practically no teaching'. His job was to do research and graduate training. The 'routine is very simple, coming in the morning and staying as long as the experiments require'. But the weekends were spent at home. He ends by saying: 'I have practically no hobbies except the family and work, which sounds somewhat dull but is not.'

Early in 1956 he was approached by the University of Basel with the suggestion that he might succeed Professor Verzar who was retiring from the Chair of Physiology, but he was well settled in the United States and it is hardly surprising that he did not pursue the matter. This was not the only approach: in November 1958 the question was mooted whether he would be interested in succeeding W. O. Fenn in Physiology at Rochester, N.Y. Kuffler's reply was non-committal, he clearly did not want to chair a big department with heavy administrative and teaching responsibilities. Nevertheless, with his rapidly growing international stature, the requests from intending postdoctoral visitors and the pressure on laboratory space increased, so much that 'by the middle 1950s the place became unbelievably crowded with capable and productive young people. This state of affairs was noticed by Harvard Medical School and they offered us space and opportunities.'

Some of Stephen's colleagues at Hopkins felt that there would have been no great difficulty in giving him all the space and facilities he required had he asked for them. But apart from this, there may have been other attractions which induced him to make a move, such as the powerful concentration of scientific activity and of excellent students at Harvard and M.I.T. and, perhaps even more important, the proximity to

Woods Hole. Anyway, by 1958–59 he felt that Harvard Medical School, on the initiative of Professor Otto Krayer, were making him 'an offer which he could not refuse'. So, in June 1959, 'about ten of us migrated to Massachusetts'. They included Torsten Wiesel, David Hubel, Edwin Furshpan, David Potter and, last but not least, R. B. Bosler who looked after the technical needs with great efficiency and held himself responsible for maintaining and continuously improving the high-class electronic apparatus which was such a vital asset and indeed indispensable for the success of Stephen's experimental work. Shortly after their arrival in Boston they were joined by E. A. Kravitz.

For over 20 years, until his death in 1980, Stephen Kuffler remained at his post at Harvard Medical School. The names attached to his appointment, and the administrative duties associated with it, changed in the course of time. He had been invited by Otto Krayer to come as Professor of Neurophysiology and Neuropharmacology and thus to add a powerful group to the Department of Pharmacology which had already under Krayer's direction established itself as one of the leading institutions in the field. In 1964 the name of Mr Robert Winthrop, a well-known benefactor was added to the professorship, but Stephen and his group remained in the Department of Pharmacology until Otto Krayer's retirement. It was, in effect, a gradually spreading sub-department devoted to a study of the nervous system, with a strong tendency to become 'multidisciplinary', going beyond the electrophysiological approach and adding the techniques of biochemistry and electron microscopy to its arsenal. In 1966, Harvard Medical School decided to establish the group formally as a Department of Neurobiology with Stephen as Chairman. He kept this position for the next 8 years, but in 1974 decided to relinquish the administrative duties associated with the running of the increasingly large department and became John F. Enders University Professor, a position which enabled him to devote his efforts entirely to research without imposing any physical changes, in facilities or location on him. This was, of course, due in no small measure to the great personal support which he received from his friends, in particular from Torsten Wiesel who had taken on the administrative headship of the department in 1974.

The strength and influence of Kuffler's Neurobiology Department was recognized internationally, and not only by those who read the publications and who received the famous annual cartoons and Christmas cards which depicted the growing membership of the group. It attracted a constant stream of young postdoctoral collaborators some of them working closely with Stephen for several years. Its fields covered neurochemistry and fine structure and later on began to extend to genetics and immunochemistry. It became a unique and leading institution and, due to the teaching and research activities of its members at the 'summer residences' of Woods Hole and the Salk Institute, its influence extended far beyond the confines of Harvard Medical School.

Stephen Kuffler and his family had settled happily in America, and since 1946 all his research work was accomplished at different laboratories in the United States. He became naturalized in 1954 and undertook various public duties, as a consultant to the Public Health Service and to the U.S. Army, as a Trustee of the Marine Biological Laboratory and as editor of physiological journals. He did also a great deal of travelling overseas, attending conferences, international congresses, honorary degree ceremonies and giving courses of lectures. It started in 1949 when he attended some of the first European postwar symposia in Madrid and Paris; in 1956, on a Guggenheim Fellowship, he took the whole family plus motor car to England and spent several months as a visitor at University College London. Later there were many more trips, to Europe, Japan, India, Australia and South America, but mostly only for quite short periods without ever seriously interrupting the research work at his home base.

The first indication of his illness came in November 1957 when he was being tested medically for some job with the U.S. Civil Service and signs of glaucoma were detected. I have mentioned the succession of medical problems and operations which afflicted Stephen without his letting them stop his work or even his holiday occupations. He continued to play tennis and to go for long swims from his Woods Hole home until the very end, and he still enjoyed travelling abroad. On his last visit to Europe, in the summer of 1980, he had a very busy schedule, receiving an honorary degree at Oxford, going on to Paris and then to Munich to give a Heisenberg lecture, attending the International Physiological Congress in Budapest and visiting Vienna on the return journey to Boston and Woods Hole, where he continued with his latest work.

There had been incidents which caused his family and friends great anxiety: Stephen had adopted a routine of self-administering insulin in the morning and following it with a regular intake of glucose to prevent his becoming hypoglycaemic during the day's work. At times this did not suffice, and there were dangerous episodes when he lapsed into unconsciousness. On one occasion he was discovered by his friends who had been alarmed because he failed to turn up for his lecture. On 11 October 1980, after his accustomed long swim in Buzzards Bay, he felt unusually exhausted and later that day died from a massive heart attack. He was buried at the place he had chosen, in a green field in Woods Hole. A Memorial Meeting was held at Harvard University Memorial Church on 3 April 1981.

Stephen Kuffler was a very fortunate person: he had a very full and happy life, his work was his main hobby and he died in the midst of it. He had received many honours and awards from the scientific community, who treasured him not only for his work, but as a warm-hearted friendly person with quite unquenchable, sometimes even mischievous sense of humour. He was always ready to demolish pretentious nonsense and to deflate pomposity wherever he detected it. The photograph reproduced [on page 142] is excellent and shows the almost irrepressible humorous glint in his eye. He liked to poke fun at himself, and he had a special knack of defusing tense situations by making them appear ridiculous before any harm was done. On occasions, he showed a 'chaplinesque' way of dispersing solemnity into a joke: for example, having just been given a flowery introduction to a formal lecture, he pretended to embrace the chairman who was about to attach the microphone round his neck, thus making it appear that he was at a ceremony receiving a most-coveted decoration! At times Stephen Kuffler tended to exasperate his friends, by appearing not to take them seriously and by turning away with a joke or a pun their attempts to raise deeply felt issues; some were critical of what seemed to them an aloofness from political issues and a reluctance to discuss controversial matters. In fact, however, he was a most generous person and very much concerned about others; if he avoided long arguments and disputes, it was because he was conscious that 'life is short', that there was not too much time left for him and most of it he wanted to keep for his top priority, which was his work.

RESEARCH WORK
Australia, 1940–45

Kuffler's first 2 years at the Sydney laboratory were a period of apprenticeship in neuromuscular research, an introduction to the technique of electric recording from cat and frog muscles, to the differences between local depolarizations in the muscle fibre, such as the 'endplate potential' set up in the region of synaptic contact by a nerve impulse, and propagated action potentials ('spikes') which, once initiated at the endplate, travel without fading to the ends of the fibre. He also found himself buffeted by continuing arguments about the role of acetylcholine as chemical mediator in the process of neuromuscular transmission and the somewhat mythical concept of a direct 'detonator' action by the nerve impulse which lingers on in one of the joint papers with J. C. Eccles (4), though its experimental foundations had all but vanished by then.

1. *The isolated nerve-muscle junction*
There is little to be said, from Kuffler's point of view, about the first half dozen joint papers in his list of publications, beyond his own comments that he did not feel very happy about his personal contributions until he took time off, at Eccles's suggestion, to learn how to isolate frog muscle fibres and for the first time to prepare an isolated nerve-muscle junction. With this he succeeded remarkably well in April 1941, and a month later sent off his first independent paper to *Nature*; the

118

full version was published in the *Journal of Neurophysiology* in 1942 (with a printer's error antedating the receipt by 1 year). This work was a brilliant technical feat, and it immediately and deservedly put him 'on the map'. The paper showed—much more clearly than had been done before—that between the arrival of a motor nerve impulse and the start of a muscle impulse there is an indispensable intermediate step in the form of a local depolarization of the muscle fibre which from previous work was known as the 'endplate potential' (e.p.p.). The experiments left little or no credibility for the 'detonator' concept according to which a muscle impulse could be initiated by the nerve action currents without intermediate local depolarization.

Kuffler used an interesting method of recording which had a number of technical advantages and some flaws: the muscle fibre with its end-plate area was kept in a bath of Ringer's solution, but the region from which he recorded rested on a fine platinum wire embedded in a glass hook and was pushed up against a layer of liquid paraffin. The other recording electrode was a wire in the large Ringer bath. It is clear from Kuffler's interpretation that he did not, at that time, fully appreciate that this method effectively records the potential difference between closely adjacent points of the fibre surface, at the exposed top of the platinum wire and the edges of the glass rod, separated from one another by approximately 0·1 mm. This 'differential' method of recording results in a wave form that approximates to the time course of the local electric *currents* as they enter into, or emerge from, the activated region of the muscle fibre, but they do not correspond directly to the local membrane *potential* change, and some of Kuffler's conclusions, regarding the height of the endplate potential and its supposed equality with the muscle spike, were subsequently found to be mistaken.

During the next 3 years, Kuffler went on to improve and exploit his isolated synaptic preparation and published a series of papers which added quantitative details and clarified previous information on nerve-muscle transmission. He studied the changes of the e.p.p. during the refractory period left behind by a previous nerve or directly initiated muscle impulse. He made experiments on the interaction between the neural transmitter and the muscle spike in normal and partly curarized fibres. He examined the depolarizing action of locally applied acetylcholine and confirmed the large and selective sensitivity to this substance of the junctional region of the muscle fibre. He also measured the increase of acetylcholine sensitivity of chronically denervated muscles, but his method of local application, with a droplet covering 2 mm of fibre length, did not allow him to discriminate between endplate and 'extrajunctional' receptors. The important fact that supersensitivity of denervated muscle is due to a spatial spread of receptors along the fibres rather than a local change at the junctional site was only established later in other laboratories.

119

He studied the different actions of calcium and calcium deficiency on nerve-muscle transmission and in further experiments produced artificial tetany in frogs and cats by surgical removal of the parathyroid glands. There were several other contributions on the single fibre dealing with the actions of veratrine and re-examining the question of whether the local electric excitability of the endplate differs from the rest of the muscle fibre.

As was to be expected, the use of such a uniquely suitable preparation helped to produce much more clear-cut and convincing evidence than was previously available. But a large part was a confirmation of existing ideas, and there were a number of weak points in this early work of which Kuffler was very conscious later on. Thus, there is an inexplicable erroneous statement in the 1943 paper on the 'specific excitability of the endplate region' (10), namely that local potassium application gave rise to impulses only at the endplate, a conclusion which he later corrected (see paper 17), and there are some doubts also about the quantitative effects ascribed to caffeine in paper 10. In retrospect, one also wonders how, in his experiments on the interaction between directly excited muscle spike and nerve-released transmitter, Kuffler missed the important finding that the e.p.p. can interfere with and substantially reduce the peak of the action potential. This observation which provided important clues to the ionic mechanism of the transmitter action was left to others several years later. One can only guess why Stephen failed to see it; perhaps he did not choose optimal time intervals for this effect, or he worked under conditions of less than optimal acetylcholine release which might have made the change too small to attract his attention.

It has sometimes been claimed that the electrophysiological work on the single neuromuscular junction was decisive in establishing the role of acetylcholine as the transmitter, but this is quite unrealistic and was certainly not the view taken by Stephen Kuffler himself. In a letter to Otto Loewi, dated May 1948, he wrote: 'On the whole my story has not contributed anything new to the well known notion that conduction along the axons is different from transmission across the junction.' The fact is that chemical mediation by acetylcholine at the neuromuscular junction had been established by the experiments of H. H. Dale, W. Feldberg, Marthe Vogt and G. L. Brown in the 1930s. Later on, the application of electrophysiological microtechniques with their special resolving powers for brief localized events was able to throw much light on detailed aspects of the process without fundamentally altering the basic proposition. It is of course true that a novel concept like the acetylcholine story needed many years to sink in, and that all kinds of objections were raised, even after Stephen's work, on premises which did not stand up to further tests. But while the strength of the original theory may have been enhanced in the eyes of those who, following Karl Popper, tried and failed to 'falsify' it, the unsuccessful 'falsifiers' can hardly claim very much credit for it.

2. *Applied electromyography*

There were two other lines of research pursued by Kuffler during his Sydney period: these were human electromyography and its clinical applications, in conjunction with Major A. M. Harvey, and, later, a study of the crustacean muscle system with its antagonistic, excitatory and inhibitory nerve supply, in which I collaborated with him.

Harvey and Kuffler developed a simple method of recording action potentials of human limb muscles in response to electric stimulation of the motor nerve, and using it to assess the extent of lesions and recovery in the peripheral nerve-muscle system (papers 11, 12, 14, 15).

3. *Nerve-muscle transmission in Crustacea*

The work on neuromuscular transmission in Crustacea concentrated on a number of features by which this system differed from that of vertebrates. Apart from the presence of a peripheral inhibitory nerve supply, and the very pronounced facilitation of the muscle response during repetitive stimulation, the most important difference is that contraction of crustacean muscle can be initiated and activated to a large extent via local non-propagated potential changes which are analogous to the e.p.p. At high frequencies of stimulation, full-size action potentials which are capable of propagation can also be elicited in some of the muscle fibres. But in contrast to vertebrate muscles, these spikes are a supplementary and not the principal mechanism for the activation of contraction, intensifying the process without being essential (moreover, crustacean muscle action potentials are now known to be 'calcium' rather than 'sodium' spikes). To a large extent, these experiments supported the views of Wiersma and van Harreveld who had obtained evidence that the activity of crustacean muscle fibres was graded, and not of the all-or-none type encountered in the vertebrates. In particular, neuromuscular facilitation in Crustacea arises mainly from a progressive increase in the amplitude of the local 'e.p.ps' and not from all-or-none recruitment of additional whole muscle fibres.

These experiments also provided a strong indication that depolarization of the muscle fibre membrane is directly related in a quantitative manner to activation of contraction in the interior of the cell. This relation was studied in more detail by Kuffler on isolated muscle fibres of the frog subjected to various electrical and chemical agents which initiate local contractures (paper 19). In every case, activation of the contractile process required depolarization of the fibre surface. When the local potential change exceeded a certain 'threshold' level, the fibre began to contract in that region, and the strength and duration of the mechanical response were graded and varied with the size of the depolarization. A particularly striking observation was that any local contraction, induced by the application of potassium or a depolarizing drug, could be made to relax promptly by electrically repolarizing the fibre surface.

121

A second paper on crustacean muscle dealt with the response to inhibitory nerve impulses. Marmont and Wiersma had made the interesting observation that, depending on the times of arrival of inhibitory and motor impulses, the former can stop the contraction without interfering with the electrical response of the muscle, that is without reducing the size of the e.p.p. Kuffler and I confirmed this observation, though later work suggests that our method of extracellular recording from the whole muscle was inadequate and failed to reveal a significant shortening of the e.p.ps. This would be quite enough to explain the apparent paradox, for it would mean that the maintained average depolarization of the muscle fibres, during repetitive nerve activity, would decrease substantially. When the inhibitory impulses arrived a few milliseconds *before* the start of each e.p.p., then the amplitude of the latter did become greatly reduced. We wrongly attributed this effect to a 'curare-like' action of the inhibitory transmitter on the postsynaptic receptors. As was shown later by Dudel and Kuffler, it arises from a separate process of 'presynaptic inhibition', that is an interference by the inhibitory transmitter with the activation of the motor nerve endings and their ability to release the normal quantity of excitatory transmitter substance. In short, the 1945 work on synaptic inhibition in crustacean muscle was merely an interesting forerunner of later work done with intracellular recording technique, and its conclusions needed drastic revision.

Chicago, 1945–47

4. *The 'slow muscles' of the frog*

When Stephen arrived in Chicago, R. W. Gerard drew his attention to a paper by Tasaki and Mizutani which suggested that the discarded hypothesis of a separate system of 'tonic' muscle fibres (i.e. non-propagating elements which contract and relax very slowly) may after all have some substance. Since he had recently encountered a somewhat similar system in Crustacea, the idea of pursuing the matter in vertebrates must have appealed to Stephen, and he chose a suitable frog muscle, the *extensor longus* of the fourth toe, for this purpose. In a preliminary paper (22), he reported two types of muscle response to stimulation of a group of small motor axons, one consisting of small local e.p.ps of slow time course associated with barely visible movement, but which summated effectively during repetitive nerve impulses to build up a strong local contraction. The other response was the typical propagated muscle spike accompanied by a fast twitch. In his first paper, Kuffler was evidently thinking in terms of the crustacean analogy; he suggested that both types of response occurred in the same muscle fibre and could be elicited by different rates of stimulation of a single small nerve axon, whereas a large axon would only evoke the propagated response. In the full paper (24) published a year later, doubts are expressed about this interpretation, and the question of a dual type of response and of innervation in a *single* muscle fibre is left open. The matter was settled several years later, by Kuffler and Vaughan Williams (and reinforced by the work of Burke and Ginsborg), showing unequivocally that two quite separate nerve-muscle fibre systems exist side-by-side, each giving only one type of response: (i) large motor axons supplying propagating twitch fibres, and (ii) multiple small axons connected to non-propagating slow fibres. Moreover, the two types of muscle fibre have different histological and ultrastructural appearance.

The small nerve axons of the 'slow' system have a relatively high threshold when tested with electric stimuli, but the normal reflex activation of their spinal neurons occurs at quite a low level of sensory stimulation and, in fact, slow muscle fibres show a great deal of 'spontaneous' background activity in spinal preparations. It is a system peculiar to the frog and well suited for the maintenance of prolonged slow contractions; the old idea of a separate type of 'tonic' muscle response useful for holding operations and posture was thus resuscitated in quite an unmistakable fashion.

The immediate reaction when the paper was submitted to the *Journal of Neurophysiology* was a letter dated 9 March 1947 from John Fulton, its chief editor, saying

> 'We do not believe that the work is well controlled and we are fearful that you are bringing up once again the old red herring of dual innervation which did so much to retard the progress of neurophysiology after the last war.'!!

Professor J. F. Fulton was a recognized authority in the field of neurophysiology, well known for his textbooks and not prepared to tolerate contradictions to what he considered established physiological principles. He had already been engaged for 10 years in a struggle against the chemical transmission theory, and was not now going to put up with the suggestion that muscle tone could be due to anything other than the classical type of impulses. However, in spite of this rather pompous editorial condemnation, it did not take very long before the conclusions of the paper were accepted by all physiologists; in fact the paper did appear in the same year, and I do not suppose that Stephen had any further trouble from this source.

Baltimore, 1947–59

During his 12 years at the Wilmer Institute of Ophthalmology at Johns Hopkins Medical School, Kuffler made some outstanding contributions to neurophysiology, whose importance was matched by their technical elegance. The highlights were the very influential work on 'concentric' receptive field arrangements of retinal ganglion cells, done with a superb *in situ* technique in the mammalian retina, and the study—with C. Eyzaguirre—of synaptic inhibition in the crustacean stretch receptor neuron, some of whose records decorate most modern neurophysiological textbooks. There were also the important further experiments, with E. M. Vaughan-Williams, on the slow-fibre system of the frog, and the investigations, with C. C. Hunt, of the intrafusal motor system in the cat.

5. *More on neuromuscular transmitter action*

But before applying himself to these new tasks, Stephen returned for a short time to the old problems of the neuromuscular junction in preparation for a special symposium paper he was to present at the 1948 Federation Meetings at Atlantic City. This paper is of historical, rather than scientific interest, in that it illustrates the perennial antagonism towards the chemical transmission concept which still seemed to be dominant at that time in Stephen's scientific environment. He reported some new experiments in which he showed that there was an irreducible delay between the moment of excitation of the prejunctional nerve twigs and the start of the e.p.p., amounting to about 1 ms in the frog at 20 °C. This was indeed difficult to reconcile with the basic postulate of electric transmission, namely that the currents produced by the nerve impulse could spread directly to the muscle fibre and excite it. It therefore gave indirect support to the acetylcholine hypothesis. However, the main body of the paper is devoted to a long argument about the nature of the agent by which the nerve impulse sets up an e.p.p., and I remember at the time being struck by what seemed to me an attitude of bending over backwards to an extent that must have been painful. In our papers on the effects of curare and eserine in 1941–42, our consensus had been that, without making unreasonable assumptions, all our observations were compatible 'with the hypothesis that acetylcholine is responsible for all the potential changes set up by nerve impulses'. But in the meantime J. C. Eccles had reconsidered the matter, and as late as 1946 he was still fighting a rearguard action against the acetylcholine story at the nerve-muscle junction. Moreover, some of the most prominent neurophysiologists in the United States remained highly sceptical about the chemical trans-mission ('soup-versus-spark') concept, and clearly did not appreciate the weight of the evidence (or perhaps refused to read the papers) on which it was based. Under these circumstances, it is no wonder that Stephen was extremely cautious in discussing the pros and cons of electrical versus chemical transmission, though even then I felt that his time could have been more usefully employed, and it was rather irritating to see him put the word transmitter in inverted commas whenever he used it, and the final conclusion regarding the nature of the 'transmitter' to read like this: 'It is thought that ions liberated during the "breakdown" in the nerve terminals could best account for the observed phenomena'!

6. The intrafusal motor system in the cat

The work in Chicago had shown the existence in the frog of a system of small motor axons which produced a 'tonic' type of contraction unaccompanied by propagated muscle spikes. After that, it became important to find out whether a similar system was also present in mammals. Suggestions of this kind had appeared from time to time, but when Kuffler and Hunt investigated the matter in the cat, they found a very different situation. Confirming and extending earlier observations by B. H. C. Matthews in 1933 and by L. Leksell in 1945, they showed that stimulation of the small diameter axons in the ventral roots of the cat caused no visible muscle contraction, but gave rise to an increased rate of firing of sensory impulses originating in the muscle spindles, presumably via activation of intrafusal muscle fibres. The experiments were done by separating spinal nerve roots into small fibre bundles which made it possible to stimulate single small axons in the ventral root (supplying a particular muscle) and to record impulses from a single dorsal root axon which originate in a spindle of the same muscle. Thus, while there is a clear division between large and small motor axons in the frog as well as the cat, the small axons serve different functions in the two animals. In the frog, the small nerve fibres supply a slowly contracting, 'non-propagating' set of muscle fibres, whereas in the cat they serve to 'pre-stretch' and thereby increase the mechanical sensitivity of the muscular 'strain gauges'. (Incidentally, the frog also possesses an efferent motor system for activating its intrafusal muscle fibres, but it is done in a 'cheap' way through branches of the ordinary motor axons; hence, adjustments of the spindle 'bias' occur merely as an accompaniment of general muscle activity. Unlike the cat, the frog does not possess a separate reflex system for controlling its spindle sensitivity.)

7. Retinal receptive fields and 'lateral inhibition'

Stephen Kuffler's incursion into retinal physiology might have been regarded simply as an outcome of his appointment at an ophthalmological institution. There is no doubt that the help and advice given by Dr. S. A. Talbot was instrumental in promoting these experiments. Talbot had designed a multibeam ophthalmoscope which enabled Kuffler to record impulses from single retinal ganglion cells under ophthalmoscopic control of the electrode position and of the stimulating light spots in an otherwise intact cat's eye. Stephen Kuffler was not particularly interested in problems of photo-reception or the sensory cells of the retina. He was using the optic neurons as a suitably accessible outpost of the brain and wanted to study the interaction of excitatory and inhibitory influences on a central nerve cell, further pursuing the problems he had been investigating previously in the crustacean neuromuscular system. His particular object was to examine the limitations and sharpness of the 'receptive field' of the cat retinal ganglion cells, building on earlier observations by H. K. Hartline. He found that each neuron responded to light spots falling on a discrete circular field of the retina, one or a few millimetres in diameter, but the responses were of opposite kind depending on whether the light impinged on the central area or the peripheral fringe of the field. If in any one neuron, illumination of the centre produced 'excitation' (i.e. an increased rate of impulse discharge), illumination of the peripheral fringe caused a reduction or stoppage of impulse activity (i.e. 'inhibition'). In other neurons these effects were reversed, that is light spots inhibited the neuron if they impinged on the centre of the field, and excited if they fell on the periphery. This type of functional organization in which converging influences from many retinal receptors and intermediate cells interact renders an assembly of optic neurons highly sensitive to the movement of a small object across the visual field, and in particular it will serve to enhance the 'contrast' between adjacent areas of different light intensity. This was pioneering work which must have influenced the research on the functional organization of the visual cortex pursued subsequently in Kuffler's department by his colleagues Hubel and Wiesel. It should be noted that quite independently similar results had been obtained at the same time by H. B. Barlow who was studying the organization of the receptive fields of frog retinal ganglion cells. A few years after this work was done, Barlow joined Kuffler's laboratory, and together with R. Fitzhugh they published a series of papers on various special aspects arising from the earlier study, in particular on the continuous spontaneous firing of optic neurons in complete darkness, and on the changes in visual threshold and the alterations in the size and organization of the receptive fields during dark adaptation. One gets the impression that these subjects were of more immediate interest to his colleagues than to Stephen himself, who by that time had gone on to look for other preparations and for more direct techniques to study the interaction of excitatory and inhibitory synapses on single nerve cells.

8. *The crustacean stretch receptor neuron and synaptic inhibition*

He found a most suitable experimental object in the large sensory neurons in the lobster and crayfish 'tail' muscles. These are stretch receptors, natural strain gauges like the muscle spindles of vertebrates. Their structure and pattern of innervation had been well described by J. S. Alexandrowicz, and their sensory function had been shown by Wiersma and his collaborators. Kuffler was joined in the course of this research by C. Eyzaguirre. Most of the experiments on Crustacea were made in the Woods Hole laboratory where there was a plentiful supply of splendid specimens which were found useful for experimental as well as culinary purposes.

The crustacean stretch receptor neuron with its various sensory and 'modulatory' synaptic connections presents an intriguing miniature nervous system on its own, and thanks to its large size, the cell body, axon and dendrites and the influence of regulatory impulses in the axons supplying the attached strand of muscle fibres, and in the inhibitory nerve fibre contacting the receptor neuron, all these can be studied directly with micro-recording techniques. The outstanding feature of the series of papers that Kuffler and Eyzaguirre published are the beautiful records which illustrate in a most impressive manner the sensory 'generator potential', that is the local depolarization set up in the dendrites of the receptor neuron by stretch or contractile activation of the attached muscle fibres, and the potentials due to stimulation of the inhibitory axon. These tend to 're-polarize' the neuronal membrane and hold it at or near its resting potential well below the firing level at which sensory impulses are initiated and discharged along the axon process. The quantitative relation between generator potential and impulse frequency, the process of adaptation, the site of origin of propagated impulse activity, the membrane conductance change during inhibition and the 'null-point' (or 'equilibrium level') of the inhibitory potential change, all these were measured and illustrated in a most decorative manner. Kuffler and C. Edwards further studied the action of gamma-aminobutyric acid which at that time was not yet established as the natural inhibitory transmitter, but appeared to reproduce its effects quite faithfully. Their interpretation of the ionic mechanism underlying the inhibitory process had to be revised later when it became clear that an increase of chloride rather than potassium permeability was involved. But altogether, the study on the stretch receptor neuron was one of the brilliant highlights of Kuffler's research work, and it was elegantly summarized in his Harvey Lecture delivered in March 1959.

Boston, 1959–80

9. *Presynaptic inhibition in Crustacea*

After his move to the Harvard Medical School, Kuffler continued to work on the crustacean neuromuscular system. He was joined by Dr Josef Dudel from Heidelberg, and the outcome was a series of important papers in the *Journal of Physiology*, analysing the effects of excitatory and inhibitory nerve impulses on crayfish muscle. The first two papers showed that, in spite of the different transmitter substances, the mechanism of release from the nerve endings was essentially the same as at the vertebrate nerve-muscle junction: spontaneous 'miniature e.p.ps' could be recorded which formed the quantal unit of the impulse-evoked 'junction potential'; the process of neuromuscular facilitation, although much more striking and extensive in crustacea, is due to a recruitment at each junctional site of additional quantal units, just as in vertebrates. However, the third paper by Dudel and Kuffler which dealt with the mechanism of neuromuscular inhibition disclosed something quite new, namely that the inhibitory nerve impulse, quite apart from its direct postsynaptic effect on the ionic permeability of the muscle fibre, was able to interfere with the power of the motor nerve impulse to release its normal amount of transmitter. In order to reveal the full extent of this 'presynaptic inhibition', the inhibitory impulse had to be timed accurately so as to arrive at the junction just before the excitatory impulse reached the motor nerve terminals. The effect was greatly to reduce the number of quantal packets of transmitter, and temporarily to lower the frequency of 'miniature e.p.ps' recorded in the muscle fibre. This was, in fact, the first unequivocal demonstration of a process of presynaptic inhibition, for which much evidence has been obtained subsequently in the central nervous system of vertebrates, and morphological correlates in the form of 'cascading' or 'series synapses' were soon found in the electron microscope.

10. *Gamma-aminobutyric acid (GABA)—an inhibitory transmitter in Crustacea*

Dudel and Kuffler also showed that all the effects, pre- and post-synaptic, of the inhibitory impulse could be reproduced by local application of GABA, which naturally led to the next series of experiments, in conjunction with E. Kravitz and D. Potter, on the local distribution of this substance in the crustacean nervous system.

To procure adequate material presented a logistic problem: large crates of lobsters arrived in Kuffler's laboratory, and the post-experimental orgies of crustacean meals must have reached saturation point during this period of his research. After some five hundred lobsters had been 'sacrificed' and their nervous system subjected to a long series of fractionations, ten different amino acids were found which produced inhibitory effects on the neuromuscular junction, GABA being by far the most potent among them. The work culminated in a heroic dissection exercise in the course of which single motor and inhibitor axons were isolated from a large number of animals to produce a total length of 'over 5 metres of lobster axon'. The results were well worth the trouble: the inhibitory nerve fibres were found to contain GABA at a concentration of the order of 100 mM, making up some 0.5% of their fresh mass, whereas nothing (meaning less than 1/1000 of this amount) was found in the accompanying motor axons. Although Kuffler and his collaborators expressed themselves very cautiously concerning the physiological significance of their observations, to most of us this result together with previous findings on the actions of GABA was convincing evidence for its identification as the inhibitory transmitter. This conclusion was strengthened by later work, some of it in Kuffler's laboratory, by A. and N. Takeuchi, and by M. Otsuka, L. L. Iversen, Z. W. Hall and E. A. Kravitz.

11. *Electrophysiology of glia cells*

After this surfeit of lobster axons, Stephen relinquished the field of crustacean neurophysiology. He turned instead to some entirely new and original problems, namely the physiology of glia, the 'satellite cells' which surround all neurons and their axon processes. It would be interesting to know what was the immediate cause for Kuffler's departure into this new area of research. He mentions (paper 68) that the work had been planned for over 10 years, but was not given very high priority. One possible indication was an aside in his recently published paper on the GABA content of single axons: 'one should note that the isolated fibres we analysed were still a complex tissue because the dissections left... the Schwann cell layer around the neuron membrane'. He was evidently a little worried by the perennial problem of whether one is correct in attributing determinations of physical and chemical properties to the nerve cells alone, or whether the results might be vitiated by the unavoidable presence of a glia or Schwann cell envelope. Various speculations were current at the time, ranging from those that attributed to the satellite cells a purely mechanical supporting role to those who thought they might have a trophic function or even actively participate in the process of nerve signalling. This last possibility was unequivocally ruled out by the work of Kuffler and his co-authors.

He was joined in these experiments by several colleagues, notably by D. D. Potter and R. K. Orkand, and by John Nicholls with whom he continued to collaborate closely for many years, first in the laboratory and later in preparing an outstandingly good textbook (*From neuron to brain*, 1976). The experiments were done on the central nervous system of the leech; later the optic nerves of frogs and mudpuppies were also studied. Using intracellular microtechniques, Kuffler and his colleagues could demonstrate that the nerve cells in the leech continued to conduct impulses after their investing glia cells had been removed by microsurgery. They also showed that glia cells, although electrically coupled to one another by low-resistance cytoplasmic pathways, are not linked to the neurons which they surround and do not themselves give action potentials. A very interesting and novel finding was that glia cells not only contain a high internal potassium concentration like nerve cells, but their surface membrane shows a more highly selective potassium permeability and a higher resting potential than the neurones. The glial membrane can therefore be used—like a specific potassium electrode—as a sensitive index for small changes in local potassium concentration which occur during repetitive activity of the adjacent nerve cells. Potassium ions leave the neurons during their action potentials and are reabsorbed only relatively slowly. They tend, therefore, to accumulate in the narrow extracellular clefts between active neurons and surrounding glia cells and cause a progressive depolarization of the latter which can build up to a level of many millivolts. Thus, some of the slow potential changes

129

recorded during electro-encephalography are probably due to local depolarization of glial syncytia.

The use of the glial membrane as an index of the extracellular potassium concentration enabled Kuffler and his colleagues to answer certain questions concerning ionic concentration gradients existing between the cerebral blood supply, the immediate environment of the central nerve cells and the cerebro-spinal fluid. While the concentrations of potassium in the blood and c.s.f. were known from direct determinations, the concentration around the neurons could now be measured for the first time, by electrical methods, and was found to correspond closely to that in the c.s.f. Another important observation was made when the sodium in the outside bath was replaced by iso-osmotic sucrose: within 10 s the nerve cells became inexcitable which showed that the extracellular sodium concentration had dropped quickly below the level at which an action potential could be elicited. The process was just as rapidly reversed by returning to normal sodium. The glial membrane potential remained constant throughout this procedure, which indicated that the potassium gradient (and by implication the internal ionic composition of the glia cell) had not been disturbed during the drastic extracellular concentration changes.

The work on the electrophysiology of glia cells was a very interesting and original departure, and was ably summarized by Kuffler and Nicholls in a review in *Ergebnisse der Physiologie* (73) and in Kuffler's Ferrier Lecture in 1965 (74). As they point out, the principal problem concerning the roles of satellite cells in the function of the nervous system remained 'on the table', and many tantalizing questions were left open in the absence of 'more precise information about the biochemical properties of various glial cells and about the nature of neuron-glia interaction'.

12. *Synaptic transmission in autonomic ganglia*

After his excursion into the physiology of satellite cells, Kuffler returned to the study of synapses, seeking a preparation that would allow him to make even more direct observations on single neuronal contacts. In his paper with U. J. McMahan (77) he recounts that 'we have searched for a preparation which would survive well in isolation and in which one could directly observe nerve cell bodies, their pre- and postsynaptic axons and surrounding glial or Schwann cells. We especially wanted to see the outlines of synaptic boutons on the surface of living nerve cells, which would enable us to do experiments on neuron-to-neuron synapses that have so far not been possible.' This search led them to the very thin and transparent interatrial septum of the frog's heart with the parasympathetic nerve ganglia embedded in it. By carrying out a preliminary study, using interference optics combined with electron microscopy and a variety of staining methods, they not only familiarized themselves with the fine structure of the septal neurons, but obtained the most magnificent pictures of synapses on living cells. This was followed by an experimental attack, in collaboration with M. J. Dennis and A. J. Harris, examining synaptic transmission with the usual electrophysiological microtechniques. This work provided a great deal of detailed information on the acetylcholine-mediated postsynaptic potentials, their quantal composition, the spatial distribution of acetylcholine-sensitive sites on the neuron surface, and their spread after surgical denervation. However, the physiological detail that resulted from these experiments must have come as something of an anti-climax after the beautiful structural study preceding it, for it showed little more than that the main features were very similar to what had been found at other synapses such as the neuromuscular junction.

13. *High-resolution studies on the nerve-muscle junction*

No such feeling is aroused by the next series of investigations, done in collaboration with D. Yoshikami, which mark a return of Stephen's personal attention to the neuromuscular synapse. Viewing endplates on the surface of muscles with interference contrast, and 'cleaning' the fibres with collagenase, they examined the localization of acetylcholine-sensitive sites with even finer spatial resolution that had previously been obtained. They found extremely steep gradients of drug sensitivity, falling to a level two orders of magnitude lower than at the actual synaptic contact area, when the tip of the testing micropipette was moved only 2 μm away. An even sharper decline was found in the spatial decrement of cholinesterase activity when this was examined by ionophoretic application of an esterase inhibitor. This work was followed by a paper with H. C. Hartzell and D. Yoshikami in which they showed an interesting interaction occurring during the release of multiple packets of acetylcholine at a single endplate: normally, the effects of the large number of individual packets, which are discharged by a single nerve impulse at hundreds of adjacent sites, are confined to a very small membrane area and do not interact, because the acetylcholine is rapidly hydrolysed near the site of its release and initial action. But when the esterase has been inhibited, the transmitter can diffuse laterally to adjacent sites and, because of the nonlinear, 'co-operative' summation of its fringe effects, interaction now occurs and leads to a very marked prolongation of the endplate potential.

The most important piece of this series is the last paper by Kuffler and Yoshikami in which they describe a technique of quantitatively assaying the amounts of acetylcholine discharged electrically from a micropipette onto an endplate. This was done by injecting acetylcholine ionophoretically with a series of recorded pulses into a measured droplet of Ringer solution and comparing its depolarizing effect on a given endplate with that of similar droplets containing various known acetylcholine concentrations. The aim of the paper was to obtain an improved estimate of the minimum amount of acetylcholine needed to reproduce a miniature endplate potential, in other words to get a better idea of the acetylcholine-equivalent of the quantal packet delivered by the nerve. The answer was that, with the pipette placed in an optimal position, very close to the most sensitive spots of the endplate, rather less than 10 000 molecules of acetylcholine had to be discharged to produce a response equivalent to a m.e.p.p. This result was of importance in connection with the 'vesicular hypothesis', i.e. that the presynaptic vesicles seen in the electron microscope are the containers of the quantal packet of acetylcholine, and are able to discharge their soluble contents in an all-or-none manner into the synaptic cleft, by a process of membrane fusion and 'exocytosis'. Previous estimates of the number of acetylcholine molecules needed to produce a quantal response had been much higher and made it difficult to believe that such an amount could be accommodated within a 50 nm vesicle. Kuffler and Yoshikami's results removed this objection.

14. *Slow synaptic potentials and a new transmitter substance*

Kuffler's last researches were devoted to a study of slow synaptic effects recorded in a variety of autonomic ganglia of the frog and mudpuppy. It had long been known that the same transmitter, acetylcholine, can produce very different effects at different synapses. The response may be a depolarization leading to an impulse, or an inhibitory change of ion conductance which stabilizes the membrane potential and prevents the initiation of an impulse in the postsynaptic cell. The effects may also differ in their time course, and in the synaptic latency before the response becomes visible; the latter can vary over more than three orders of magnitude. The fast responses at the motor endplate are presumably due to a direct action of the transmitter, and cease when the acetylcholine molecules dissociate from the membrane receptors. Kuffler and his colleagues (87) studied an additional inhibitory action of acetylcholine in a parasympathetic neuron, which had a much slower onset and longer duration. This late response arose well after the acetylcholine had exerted its brief excitatory action on the same neuron, and presumably long after it had diffused away. There were some characteristic pharmacological differences between the brief and slow responses, indicating that the acetylcholine acted on two different kinds of membrane receptors, the so-called 'nicotinic' and 'muscarinic' types. While the fast nicotinic response may well be due to a direct action of the transmitter itself, the muscarinic response seems to occur only at the end of an intermediate sequence of chemical reaction steps.

Finally, in conjunction with Drs Y. N. and L. Y. Jan, Kuffler made the important discovery of a peptide-operated synapse in sympathetic ganglia of the frog. In his last paper, in a publication of a symposium that was held in his honour at Woods Hole in April 1980, he describes 'events in sympathetic ganglia . . . where release of acetylcholine initiates three different synaptic potentials: (i) a standard fast nicotinic e.p.s.p. (about 30–50 ms duration); (ii) a slow muscarinic e.p.s.p. (30–60 s); (iii) a slow i.p.s.p. (about 2 s). The fourth synaptic signal, the "late slow e.p.s.p.", lasts 5–10 min and is not caused by acetylcholine. We have evidence that a peptide, resembling luteinizing hormone releasing hormone (LHRH), is secreted by specific axons within ganglia where it initiates the late slow e.p.s.ps.' He then recounts the several lines of chemical as well as electrophysiological experiments which led to this conclusion (intraneuronal detection of a peptide of appropriate molecular weight by radioimmunoassay; detection of its calcium-dependent release in high potassium media; disappearance of peptide after denervation; evidence for its production in the neuron and transport along the axon; characteristic postsynaptic effect of direct LHRH application; specific blocking action of impulse-evoked response by a LHRH antagonist). In the summer of 1980, Stephen Kuffler gave a full report on this work to the International Physiological Congress at Budapest; his lecture was regarded as one of the outstanding highlights of this Congress. Immediately afterwards he returned to Woods Hole, and was actively engaged together with Dr T. Sejnowski in experiments designed to elucidate further the mechanism of postsynaptic action of LHRH. He died in the midst of these activities.

Stephen Kuffler had the good fortune to find endless excitement in his life's work. In the course of it he made many important discoveries and brought new light to many areas of neurobiology. His work adds up to a magnificent volume of physiological research; his experimental results were usually accompanied by beautiful illustrations, which added clarity and gave much pleasure to his readers. Technical accomplishment was one of the outstanding features of his research, but he always used his technical skill for a definite purpose, namely to obtain experimental results which were simple and capable of straightforward interpretation, and in this way could give a clear answer to a scientific question. Theory was not his particular line, nor the development of a grand new concept. What he wanted to achieve was to reveal the inherent beauty of the detailed mechanisms whereby nerve cells go about their daily business. In his experimental pursuits he had the gift of making an almost unerring choice of the most suitable living preparation: in this he seems to have emulated one of his scientific heroes, Ramon y Cajal, whom he describes (86) as 'one of the greatest students of the nervous system, selecting samples from a wide range of the animal kingdom with an almost unfailing instinct for the essential'.

I have been greatly helped in the preparation of this memoir by Dr Phyllis Kuffler, Mrs Margaret Wilmot and Professor Felix Mlczoch who gave me important information about Stephen Kuffler's life in Hungary and Austria, and I am indebted for much valuable assistance to Mrs Marion Kozodoy and Professor Torsten Wiesel. The photograph is by Fabian Bachrach, Boston.

APPENDIX I

(a) *Honorary degrees*

1959   M.A. Harvard University
1964   M.D. University of Bern, Switzerland
1972   D.Sc. Yale University
1974   D.Sc. Washington University, St. Louis
1974   D.Sc. University of London
1977   D.Sc. University of Chicago
1977   D.Sc. Pierre and Marie Curie University (University of Paris)
1980   D.Sc. University of Oxford

(b) *Membership*

National Academy of Sciences
American Academy of Arts and Sciences
The Royal Society (Foreign Member)
Royal Danish Academy of Sciences and Letters (Foreign Member)
Austrian Academy of Sciences (Foreign Member)
Physiological Society (London)
American Physiological Society
American Philosophical Society
Bavarian Academy of Sciences (Foreign Member)

(c) *Awards and Special Lectureships*

1957, 1980   Bishop Lecturer (Washington University, St Louis)
1959   Harvey Lecturer
1965   Ferrier Lecturer (Royal Society, London)
1971   Silliman Memorial Lecturer (Yale University)
1971   Passano Award
1972   Sherrington Lecturer (Liverpool University)
1972   Louisa Gross Horwitz Prize in Biology
1973   Proctor Award in Ophthalmology
1973   Dickson Prize in Medicine
1976   Wakeman Award
1977   Armin von Tschermak-Seysenegg Prize (Austrian Academy of Sciences)
1978   Gerard Prize
1979   F. O. Schmitt Prize in Neuroscience (M.I.T.)
1979   Forbes Lecturer (Grass Foundation)
1980   Heisenberg Lecturer (Munich)

APPENDIX II

A CURRICULUM VITAE OF SORTS

By STEPHEN W. KUFFLER

[Written probably in 1971—B.K.]

I spent the first ten years of my life in Hungary on a medium-sized farm. My most vivid memories are about riding horses, swimming in ponds and occasionally visiting a near-by 'big' city. At home we spoke

Hungarian and German and learned reasonably good French from a succession of governesses. A few attempts in elementary education on a private basis by the local school teacher ended in complete failure. This existence came abruptly to an end in 1923 when I was sent to a boarding school near Vienna—a 'gymnasium' run by the Jesuits. Before they let me start on the school's eight-year course they wisely provided a year of preliminary education in order to catch up with my missing elementary schooling. After the preparatory year I stayed on for the full remaining eight years. The education was 'humanistic', with emphasis on moral rectitude of the proper sectarian variety, and eight years of Latin and six years of Greek, and practically no science.

When I finished high school in 1932, I entered medical school in Vienna, after having rejected languages and law, both of which interested me for some undefined reason. I guess I chose medicine for its international character. I spent barely more than five years in medical school, finishing my examinations during the late fall of 1937. It was a difficult and turbulent period in Austrian politics, and we had anything but a peaceful time. While I had many good friends, I strongly rejected my environment—full of violence and social unrest. I spent as little time as possible at the medical school and managed to be away a great deal. There was a period of about six months when, while still a medical student, I worked as an assistant in a hospital in the east end of London. My favourite place was the accident room, where the attending surgeon frequently let me do odd jobs. At the same time I was able to observe the local characters and learn some English. I formed a strong liking for London. Another break in my medical education was a protracted trip of tramping through the Middle East to Egypt and back again.

At the University, I was totally unprepared for the 'scientific' part of my medical courses, particularly in chemistry. This was a handicap that I have never overcome in my subsequent career. Otherwise, my main interest was pathology, which I regarded as the basis of good medicine. I may add that during my medical school years we had a total financial collapse in our family fortunes, and for long periods I made my living as a tutor of retarded high school students, at last making full use of my previous education in Greek and Latin.

On finishing medical school I began a residency in internal medicine and also worked simultaneously in the Department of Pathology in Vienna. This brief clinical exposure was terminated in March 1938, by the German invasion of Austria. Since the next war was close on the horizon and I observed the stepped up brutalities in my environment, I immediately decided to leave, hoping that the conflict would find me on the correct side. I also decided to go to an English-speaking country, preferably England. Shortly after the invasion I escaped by crossing over into Hungary and found my way to London, where I had some good friends. However, I could not use my medical qualifications and decided to apply for a visa to Australia. During my three months in England, in 1938, I had a transient non-medical job near Manchester, and I spent some time with the family of my good friends John and Charis Brophy. Brophy was a literary figure, one of the sweetest and most generous people I have ever known. We kept in close touch until 1965, when he died, but I still visit his wife Charis each time I come to London.

I bought a ticket to Brisbane, Australia—the last stop on the Orient Line, because it made practically no difference whether one got off at Perth, Adelaide, Melbourne, Sydney or at the last stop Brisbane. Anyway, I left the boat in Sydney and after two days or so of looking around, went to the university and immediately got a job as a demonstrator in pathology. This job lasted for approximately ten days or even two weeks, because in the meantime I met John Eccles who had a tennis court in his backyard, where we had a very good game. On the strength of my tennis he offered me a job as his assistant, which I accepted, not really knowing what it implied. Eccles's enthusiasm convinced me that solving the problems of one's brain, of consciousness, not to speak of such small matters as behaviour, etc. seemed a worth while task for a young man in my situation.

My work with Eccles, however, started on a much more mundane level, exploring the mysteries of the neuromuscular junction. I floundered around terribly and Eccles was extremely patient with me. After a year, in the fall of 1939, we were joined by Bernard Katz from the Department of Biophysics at University College where he had worked with A. V. Hill. We had a very fruitful few years together. The challenge of working with Eccles and Katz was almost unbearable, because both of them were so highly trained and intelligent. Since I could not compete on the intellectual plane, I took full advantage of my manual skills by preparing the first isolated nerve-muscle junction. The simplicity of that preparation compensated for my lack of sophistication, and I obtained my first independent scientific results.

The war soon disrupted the scientific collaboration between Eccles, Katz and myself. Katz and I were keen to enlist. This was easier for Katz who had become a British citizen and therefore could join the air force as a radar officer. My stint in the Australian army lasted only between thirty and sixty minutes. At the induction centre I was issued a uniform and told that I would be sent to the interior of Australia to help in road construction. This was contrary to my understanding of becoming a medical officer, preferably in the overseas forces, and I immediately claimed my status as a doctor. The refusal of the Australians to accept me in the 'proper' army was due to my being a stateless person, since I never accepted German citizenship and Austria had faded away. Anyway, the conflict was resolved by my leaving the induction station.

I had more success with the Americans, who had set up a field hospital in the Sydney area, mainly staffed by people from Johns Hopkins

University Medical School. There I functioned as a consulting neurologist working on nerve injuries that were quite plentiful in the Pacific war. These activities, however, were not full-time and I continued research work in Eccles's laboratory, even after Eccles had left for New Zealand in 1943.

Eccles's laboratory was not reconstituted after the war and Katz and I were looking for jobs. He got one at University College in biophysics, while I obtained a fellowship to go to work in Gerard's laboratory in the United States. By that time I had become a British citizen, acquired an Australian wife and one infant daughter (in 1945). I stayed in Chicago from late 1945 to early 1947, when I was offered a job in the Department of Ophthalmology, the Wilmer Institute, at Johns Hopkins Medical School.

Hopkins was a wonderful place, and they gave me a small basement laboratory that soon became filled with a group of eager young postdoctoral workers, several of them from abroad, particularly Great Britain. By the middle 1950s the place became unbelievably crowded with capable and productive young people. This state of affairs was noticed by Harvard Medical School and they offered us space and opportunities. About ten of us migrated to Massachusetts and eventually we became the founding fathers of a new Department of Neurobiology. Six of the original Hopkins group are still together, but naturally each of us has his own independent laboratory.

In 1954 I became an American citizen and have voted in every major election ever since. Our family of two boys and two girls, now successfully matured, are at the centre of my non-scientific interests. Otherwise my preoccupation remains the nervous system.

BIBLIOGRAPHY

Papers

(1) 1941 (With B. KATZ) Multiple motor innervation of the frog's sartorius muscle. *J. Neurophysiol.* **4**, 209–225.

(2) (With J. C. ECCLES & B. KATZ) Electric potential changes accompanying neuromuscular transmission. *Biol. Symp.* **3**, 349–370.

(3) (With J. C. ECCLES & B. KATZ) Nature of the 'endplate potential' in curarized muscle. *J. Neurophysiol.* **5**, 362–387.

(4) (With J. C. ECCLES) Initiation of muscle impulses at neuro-muscular junction. *J. Neurophysiol.* **4**, 402–417.

(5) (With J. C. ECCLES) The endplate potential during and after the muscle spike potential. *J. Neurophysiol.* **4**, 486–506.

(6) 1942 Electrical potential changes at an isolated nerve-muscle junction. *J. Neurophysiol.* **5**, 18–26.

(7) Responses during refractory period at myoneural junction in isolated nerve-muscle fibre preparation. *J. Neurophysiol.* **5**, 199–209.

(8) (With J. C. ECCLES & B. KATZ) Effect of eserine on neuromuscular transmission. *J. Neurophysiol.* **5**, 211–230.

(9) Further study on transmission in an isolated nerve-muscle fibre preparation. *J. Neurophysiol.* **5**, 309–322.

(10) 1943 Specific excitability of the endplate region in normal and denervated muscle. *J. Neurophysiol.* **6**, 99–110.

(11) 1944 (With A. M. HARVEY) Motor nerve function with lesions of the peripheral nerves. A quantitative study. *Archs Neurol. Psychiat., Chicago* **52**, 317–322.

(12)   (With A. M. HARVEY) Synchronization of spontaneous activity in denervated human muscle. *Archs Neurol. Psychiat., Chicago* **52**, 495–497.

(13)   The effect of calcium on the neuro-muscular junction. *J. Neurophysiol.* **7**, 17–26.

(14)   Electrical investigations in physiology and some clinical applications. *Aust. J. Sci.* **6**, 132–135.

(15) 1945 (With A. M. HARVEY & J. B. TREDWAY) Peripheral neuritis: clinical and physiological observations on a series of twenty cases of unknown etiology. *Bull. Johns Hopkins Hosp.* **77**, 83–103.

(16)   Excitability changes at the neuro-muscular junction during tetany. *J. Physiol.* **103**, 403–411.

(17)   Electric excitability of nerve-muscle fibre preparations. *J. Neurophysiol.* **8**, 77–88.

(18)   Action of veratrine on nerve-muscle preparations. *J. Neurophysiol.* **8**, 113–122.

(19) 1946 The relation of electric potential changes to contracture in skeletal muscle. *J. Neurophysiol.* **9**, 367–377.

(20)   (With B. KATZ) Excitation of the nerve-muscle system in Crustacea. *Proc. R. Soc. Lond.* B **133**, 374–389.

(21)   (With B. KATZ) Inhibition at the nerve-muscle junction in Crustacea. *J. Neurophysiol.* **9**, 337–346.

(22)   A second motor nerve system to frog skeletal muscle. *Proc. Soc. exp. Biol. Med.* **63**, 21–23.

(23) 1947 Membrane changes during excitation and inhibition of the contractile mechanism. *Ann. N.Y. Acad. Sci.* **47**, 767–779.

(24)   (With R. W. GERARD) The small-nerve motor system to skeletal muscle. *J. Neurophysiol.* **10**, 383–394.

(25)   (With Y. LAPORTE & R. E. RANSMEIER) The function of the frog's small-nerve motor system. *J. Neurophysiol.* **10**, 395–408.

(26) 1948 Physiology of neuro-muscular junctions: electrical aspects. *Fedn Proc. Fedn Am. Socs exp. Biol.* **7**, 437–446.

(27) 1949 (With C. C. HUNT) Small-nerve fibers in mammalian ventral roots. *Proc. Soc. exp. Biol. Med.* **71**, 256–257.

(28)   Transmitter mechanism at the nerve-muscle junction. *Archs Sci. physiol.* **3**, 585–601.

(29)   Le système moteur à fibres nerveuses de petit diamètre. *Archs Sci. physiol.* **3**, 613–630.

(30) 1950 (With C. C. HUNT) Pharmacology of the neuromuscular junction. *J. Pharmac. exp. Ther.* **98**, 96–120.

(31)   (With C. C. HUNT) The mammalian small-nerve fibers: a system for efferent nervous regulation of muscle spindle discharge. In: *Patterns of organization in the central nervous system*, vol. XXX, ch II, pp. 24–47. Proceedings of the Association for Research in Mental Disorders, New York, December 1950.

(32) 1951 (With C. C. HUNT & J. P. QUILLIAM) Function of medullated small-nerve fibers in mammalian ventral roots: efferent muscle spindle innervation. *J. Neurophysiol.* **14**, 29–54.

(33)   (With C. C. HUNT) Stretch receptor discharges during muscle contraction. *J. Physiol.* **113**, 298–315.

(34)   (With C. C. HUNT) Further study of efferent small-nerve fibres to mammalian muscle spindles. Multiple spindle innervation and activity during contraction. *J. Physiol.* **113**, 283–297.

(35) 1952 Transmission processes at nerve-muscle junctions. In: *Modern trends in physiology and biochemistry*, pp. 277–290. New York: Academic Press.

(36)   (With S. A. TALBOT) A multibeam ophthalmoscope for the study of retinal physiology. *J. opt. Soc. Am.* **42**, 931–936.

(37)   Neurons in the retina: organization, inhibition and excitation problems. *Cold Spring Harb. Symp. quant. Biol.* **17**, 281–292.

(38) 1953 Discharge patterns and functional organization of the mammalian retina. *J. Neurophysiol.* **16**, 37–68.

138

(39) 1953 (With E. M. VAUGHAN WILLIAMS) Small-nerve junctional potentials. The distribution of small motor nerves to frog skeletal muscle and the membrane characteristics of the fibres they innervate. *J. Physiol.* **121**, 289–317.

(40) (With E. M. VAUGHAN WILLIAMS) Properties of the 'slow' skeletal muscle fibres of the frog. *J. Physiol.* **121**, 318–340.

(41) The two skeletal nerve-muscle systems in the frog. *Arch. exper. Path. Pharmak.* **220**, 116–135.

(42) 1954 (With C. C. HUNT) Motor innervation of skeletal muscle: multiple innervation of individual muscle fibres and motor unit function. *J. Physiol.* **126**, 293–303.

(43) Mechanisms of activation and motor control of stretch receptors in lobster and crayfish. *J. Neurophysiol.* **17**, 558–574.

(44) 1955 Contractures at the nerve-muscle junction: the slow muscle fibre system. *Am. J. phys. Med.* **34**, 161–171.

(45) (With C. EYZAGUIRRE) Processes of excitation in the dendrites and in the soma of single isolated sensory nerve cells of the lobster and crayfish. *J. gen. Physiol.* **39**, 87–119.

(46) (With C. EYZAGUIRRE) Further study of soma, dendrite and axon excitation in single neurons. *J. gen. Physiol.* **39**, 121–153.

(47) (With C. EYZAGUIRRE) Synaptic inhibition in an isolated nerve cell. *J. gen. Physiol.* **39**, 155–184.

(48) 1956 (With W. TRAUTWEIN & C. EDWARDS) Changes in membrane characteristics of heart muscle during inhibition. *J. gen. Physiol.* **40**, 135–145.

(49) 1957 (With R. FITZHUGH & H. B. BARLOW) Maintained activity in the cat's retina in light and darkness. *J. gen. Physiol.* **40**, 683–702.

(50) (With H. B. BARLOW & R. FITZHUGH) Dark adaptation, absolute threshold and Purkinje shift in single units of the cat's retina. *J. Physiol.* **137**, 327–337.

(51) (With H. B. BARLOW & R. FITZHUGH) Change of organization in the receptive fields of the cat's retina during dark adaptation. *J. Physiol.* **137**, 338–354.

(52) (With A. S. V. BURGEN) Two inhibitory fibres forming synapses with a single nerve cell in the lobster. *Nature, Lond.* **180**, 1490–1491.

(53) 1958 Synaptic inhibitory mechanisms. Properties of dendrites and problems of excitation in isolated sensory nerve cells. *Expl. Cell. Res.* **5**, 493–519.

(54) (With C. EDWARDS) Mechanism of gamma aminobutyric acid (GABA) action and its relation to synaptic inhibition. *J. Neurophysiol.* **21**, 589–610.

(55) 1959 (With C. EDWARDS) The blocking effect of γ-aminobutyric acid (GABA) and the action of related compounds on single nerve cells. *J. Neurochem.* **4**, 19–30.

(56) Synaptic inhibition. *XXI Congreso Internacional de Ciencias Fisiologicas*, Buenos Aires, 9–15 August.

(57) 1960 Excitation and inhibition in single nerve cells. *The Harvey Lectures, 1958-1959*, pp. 176–218. New York: Academic Press.

(58) 1961 (With J. DUDEL) Presynaptic inhibition at the neuromuscular junction in crayfish. *Internat. Symposium 'Nervous Inhibition'* (Friday Harbor), pp. 111–113.

(59) (With J. DUDEL) The quantal nature of transmission and spontaneous miniature potentials at the crayfish neuromuscular junction. *J. Physiol.* **155**, 514–529.

(60) (With J. DUDEL) Mechanism of facilitation at the crayfish neuromuscular junction *J. Physiol.* **155**, 530–542.

(61) (With J. DUDEL) Presynaptic inhibition at the crayfish neuromuscular junction. *J. Physiol.* **155**, 543–562.

(62) 1963 (With J. DUDEL, R. GRYDER, A. KAJI & D. D. POTTER) Gamma-aminobutyric acid and other blocking compounds in Crustacea. I. Central nervous system. *J. Neurophysiol.* **26**, 721–728.

(63) (With E. A. KRAVITZ, D. D. POTTER & N. M. VAN GELDER) Gamma-aminobutyric acid and other blocking compounds in Crustacea. II. Peripheral nervous system. *J. Neurophysiol.* **26**, 729–738.

(64) (With E. A. KRAVITZ & D. D. POTTER) Gamma-aminobutyric acid and other blocking compounds in Crustacea. III. Their relative concentrations in separated motor and inhibitory axons. *J. Neurophysiol.* **26**, 739–751.

(65) 1964 (With D. D. POTTER) Glia in the leech central nervous system. Physiological properties and neuron-glia relationship. *J. Neurophysiol.*, **27**, 290–320.

(66) (With J. G. NICHOLLS) Glial cells in the central nervous system of the leech; their membrane potential and potassium content. *Arch. exp. Path. Pharmak.* **248**, 216–222.

(67) 1964 (With J. G. Nicholls) Extracellular space as a pathway for exchange between blood and neurons in the central nervous system of the leech: ionic composition of glial cells and neurons. *J. Neurophysiol.* **27**, 645–671.

(68) 1965 (With J. G. Nicholls & D. D. Potter) An approach to the study of neuroglia and of extracellular space based on recent work on the nervous system of the leech. In. *Studies in physiology* (ed. D. R. Curtis & A. K. McIntyre), pp. 152–155. Berlin: Springer-Verlag.

(69) (With J. G. Nicholls) The Na and K content of glial cells and neurons determined by flame photometry in the nervous system of the leech. *J. Neurophysiol.* **28**, 519–525.

(70) (With J. G. Nicholls) How do materials exchange between blood and nerve cells in the brain? *Perspect. Biol. Med.* **9**, 69–76,

(71) 1966 (With J. G. Nicholls & R. K. Orkand) Physiological properties of glial cells in the central nervous system of Amphibia. *J. Neurophysiol.* **29**, 768–787.

(72) (With R. K. Orkand & J. G. Nicholls) The effect of nerve impulses on the membrane potential of glial cells in the central nervous system of Amphibia. *J. Neurophysiol.* **29**, 788–806.

(73) (With J. G. Nicholls) The physiology of neuroglial cells. *Ergebn. Physiol.* **57**, 1–90.

(74) 1967 Neuroglial cells: physiological properties and a potassium mediated effect of neuronal activity on the glial membrane potential. The Ferrier Lecture. *Proc. R. Soc. Lond.* B **168**, 1–21.

(75) 1968 (With M. W. Cohen & H. M. Gerschenfeld) Ionic environment of neurones and glial cells in the brain of an amphibian. *J. Physiol.* **197**, 363–380.

(76) 1970 (With U. J. McMahan) Viewing cholinergic synaptic areas on living nerve cells of the frog's heart. In: *Excitatory synaptic mechanisms* (ed. P. Andersen & J. K. S. Jansen), pp. 57–66. Oslo: Universitetsforlaget.

(77) 1971 (With U. J. McMahan) Visual identification of synaptic boutons on living ganglion cells and of varicosities in postganglionic axons in the heart of the frog. *Proc. R. Soc. Lond.* B **177**, 485–508.

(78) (With M. J. Dennis & A. J. Harris) Synaptic transmission and its duplication by focally applied acetylcholine in para-sympathetic neurons in the heart of the frog. *Proc. R. Soc. Lond.* B **177**, 509–539.

(79) (With A. J. Harris & M. J. Dennis) Differential chemosensitivity of synaptic and extrasynaptic areas on the neuronal surface membrane in parasympathetic neurons of the frog, tested by microapplication of acetylcholine. *Proc. R. Soc. Lond.* B **177**, 541–553.

(80) (With M. J. Dennis & A. J. Harris) The development of chemosensitivity in extrasynaptic areas of the neuronal surface after deneration of parasympathetic ganglion cells in the heart of the frog. *Proc. R. Soc. Lond.* B **177**, 555–563.

(81) 1973 The single-cell approach in the visual system and the study of receptive fields. (Proctor Award Lecture, Assoc. for Res. in Vision and Ophthalmol.) *Invest. Ophthal.* **12**, 794–813.

(82) 1975 (With D. Yoshikami) The distribution of acetylcholine sensitivity at the post-synaptic membrane of vertebrate skeletal twitch muscles: iontophoretic mapping in the micron range. *J. Physiol.* **244**, 703–730.

(83) (With H. C. Hartzell & D. Yoshikami) Post-synaptic potentiation: interaction between quanta of acetylcholine at the skeletal neuromuscular synapse. *J. Physiol.* **251**, 427–463.

(84) (With D. Yoshikami) The number of transmitter molecules in a quantum: an estimate from iontophoretic application of acetylcholine at the neuromuscular synapse. *J. Physiol.* **251**, 465–482.

(85) 1976 (With H. C. Hartzell & D. Yoshikami) The number of acetylcholine molecules in a quantum and the interaction between quanta at the subsynaptic membrane of the skeletal neuromuscular synapse. *Cold Spring Harb. Symp. quant. Biol.* **40**, 175–186.

(86) (With J. G. Nicholls) *From Neuron to Brain*, pp. xiii and 486. Sunderland, Mass.: Sinauer.

(87) 1977 (With H. C. Hartzell, R. Stickgold & D. Yoshikami) Synaptic excitation and inhibition resulting from the direct action of acetylcholine on two types of chemo-receptors on individual parasympathetic neurones of an amphibian. *J. Physiol.* **271**, 817–846.

140

(88)   1979   (With Y. N. JAN & L. Y. JAN) A peptide as a possible transmitter in sympathetic ganglia of the frog. *Proc. natn. Acad. Sci. U.S.A.* **76**, 1501–1505.

(89)   1980   (With Y. N. JAN & L. Y. JAN) Further evidence for peptidergic transmission in sympathetic ganglia. *Proc. natn. Acad Sci. U.S.A.* **77**, 5008–5012.

(90)   Slow synaptic responses in autonomic ganglia and the pursuit of a peptidergic transmitter. In: *Neurotransmission, neurotransmitters, and neuromodulators* (ed. E. A. Kravitz & J. E. Treherne), *J. exp. Biol.* **89**, 257–286.

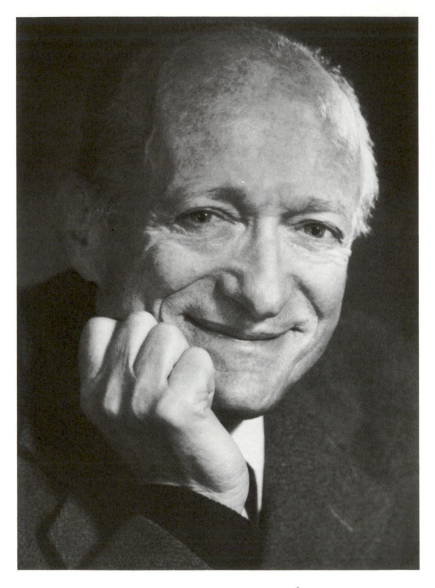